Watching EMERGENCY!
A Viewer's Off-the-Wall Guide

Seasons 1-3

May Fair

ISBN: 1981396829
ISBN-13: 978-1981396-825

This books deals with *Emergency!*, the 1970s TV show about paramedics and firefighters at the fictional Station 51, and the doctors at Rampart General's emergency department.

What this book IS NOT: This book is *not* an "official" episode guide, or an "official" anything. It doesn't discuss the background of the show or recount the history of the paramedic program. There are no "behind the scene" interviews with cast or crew, no program notes, no filming locations or listing of guest stars, writers, or directors. Such details can be found elsewhere, on fansites, media sites, Wikipedia, books, interviews, etc.

What this book IS: Instead, this book is simply the random and unprofound thoughts and comments about episodes of this fun, enjoyable show. ***The comments were originally posted on a public message board, hence the informal nature of the writing.*** For legal reasons, the entire discussions, including other users' comments, are not part of this book; with the exception of brief excerpts (quotes) provided for context, this book represents one person's views. Again, these comments were written as a "just for fun" activity and meant to be enjoyed in that context.

Some of these commentaries are more in-depth than others, and have been geared toward those who are already fans of the series. Quite a few comments mention continuity errors in the episodes; however, far from denigrating the series, these goofs actually tend to endear fans to the show all the more, so please take these comments in the (loving) spirit in which they're intended.

Episodes are reviewed at least twice here, on successive viewings over the run of the series. Follow-up comments (and replies to comments of others) are separated by a row of asterisks, and may include a brief quote. **Please note that many of the thoughts captured the first time around are touched upon again in the second review, along with 'new' insights as well. The two commentaries (old and new) are separated by a "three-peat" appearance of the tilde (~ ~ ~).

The thoughts/ideas/comments/opinions/theories expressed here belong to the writer, and are not concrete proof of anything. If those thoughts/opinions are off-the-wall, so be it, get the virtual tomatoes ready for hurling; if instead they're perceived to be brilliant, then the writer is either an extremely insightful thinker... or simply has too much time on her hands. You decide.

Main characters on the show:

Roy DeSoto – played by Kevin Tighe
John Gage – played by Randy Mantooth
Captain Stanley (Cap) – played by Mike Norell
Mike Stoker – played by Mike Stoker
Chet Kelly – played by Tim Donnelly
Marco Lopez – played by Marco Lopez
Dixie McCall – played by Julie London
Dr. Kelly Brackett – played by Robert Fuller
Dr. Joe Early – played by Bobby Troup
Dr. Mike Morton – played by Ron Pinkard

CONTENTS

Pilot Movie: The Wedsworth-Townsend Act

Whenever I watch this, I'm always surprised at the fact that the movie opens like... well, a real movie. With the studio name and everything. The Universal logo appears at the beginning, just like cinematic movies, rather than at the very end like on TV shows, when nobody actually sees it. The movie itself begins with a drawn-out view of Fire Station 10, which is crowded with a surprising number of vehicles. I guess those Chiefs' cars can't roll out on their own; they're too hemmed in by engines and other vehicles. The camera then pans up the legendary fire pole and the scene switches to the dorm, where all the good little firemen are asleep in their beds, bunker gear right next to them at the ready. Then the quiet scene is disturbed by the tones of an alarm and everyone jumps into action. Well, first they jump into their bunker boots and pants, and *then* they jump into action.

That's when we see all the equipment roll out of the station. Seriously, it was like watching a clown car with all those vehicles spilling out of that small station. And when they get to the huge fire the Battalion Chief (who's based out of that station, apparently) calls for a second alarm, directs all the engines and trucks, etc. Then the two rescue men have to put their gear on and get a FF who passed out in the building. As soon as they come out with him, the fire seems to be out, all the firemen turn off their hoses, and the chief declares it under control. Funny, it was raging wildly just ten minutes earlier.

Couple things to note about this fire: 1) I saw a number of scenes which we will see again in the series, used as stock footage. 2) Note the funky light systems for the chief's car

and even the squad. Some sort of cloverleaf of lights on top
of them, rather than the light-bar we'll see on squad 51 and
other vehicles later on. 3) As we're watching the action, in
the background the chief is talking to the dispatcher (Sam).
Sam asks about a statement for the press, and the chief
requests additional air bottles be sent out.

No sooner does a sooty (and young!) John Gage get back to
the station than the chief reminds him about the paramedic
program; of course, Johnny is not impressed, and even less
interested. Then they go off on a rescue call: an
electrocution. John and his partner race out there (his
partner was played by the same actor who played Gil, just
the other day), and Johnny takes an air tank in the snorkel to
retrieve the victim. Other than the air and some chest
compressions, the 'rescue men' don't do a heck of a lot
more than any other fireman, I don't think. Anyway, the
guy dies despite all of Brackett's efforts (and Morton's--er,
I mean Dr. Gray's). This leads to both Brackett and Johnny
using four-letter words: Doc says "d@mn it," and Johnny
says "rescue, hell."

At Rampart, we're introduced to the kindly Dr. Joe Early
who's dealing with a tricky patient--yes, you guessed it, it's
a little boy. (Have we ever seen him treat a little girl? They
always seem to be boys. Girls can be just as rambunctious
and get into as much trouble as boys, you know!) Anyway,
he extricates the quarter the boy had ingested.... and then he
picks it up and handles it! Ewwww!! But we learn that Joe
is the "best neurosurgeon in town," and in another early
episode (or maybe this movie) it's noted that he volunteers
his time at Rampart. Obviously that storyline fades away
into oblivion and Early is just another staff physician.

Anyway, now Johnny goes to headquarters to see about the
paramedic program, including a "hand-written" note
showing that Roy DeSoto, FM, writes with red crayon and

makes funny-looking capital Qs. If you watch this scene, Roy does the same thing that Officer Pete Malloy does in the pilot of Adam-12: an informative and somewhat complicated speech full of gravitas and Important Information. (He does another mini-speech like that later on, when he first shows Johnny the new squad.) Another thing I noticed about this scene (in addition to Johnny's funky watch and the spartan office, very Dragnet-ish) is that Johnny really hardly looks at Roy at all. Usually if you ask someone questions, and they're explaining something to you, you *look at* the person who's doing the explaining. I just thought that was kind of odd. And it sort of looked like the pen Johnny borrowed to sign the form was sort of green, but I think it was actually more grey. Too bad, right?

So Johnny takes the paramedic course with Marco, and an African-American guy who could grow up to be the second Brice. Or maybe it's Stoney?? Anyway once they graduate and Roy and John are assigned to the "new" station 51 they get to go on some runs. And who do they take with them? Dixie. In a pantsuit, no less. Did she change clothes from her dress to the pants before leaving the hospital? She sure never wore pants at Rampart during the first three seasons. (Or was it two? can't recall.)

The car crash they respond to.... that girl looked for all the world like Linda Kelsey, the woman who would later play Drew's wife (and she'd go on to be in Lou Grant). I'd swear it's her, but I can't find confirmation anywhere. Also, what about the driver of the 2nd car?

At Rampart, a young woman is brought after her arm is severed at a boatyard. Roy and Johnny are dispatched to find it, resulting in one of the most awkward bits of dialogue of the whole hour, when Dixie asks how far the boatyard is and Roy says "What's the difference? We'll make it closer." Ugh.

3

Oh, when they were treating the electrocution guy at the hospital and Brackett used the defibrillator on him, he asked Dixie, "Give me a reading," and she said "400 watt seconds." We get a close-up of the machine, and the dial clearly goes only up to 200 watt seconds. Am I missing something with that?

Well, part 2 tomorrow. The good news is, no Kel and Dixie kissing in that one. The bad news: the awkward party she throws, and that awful Joanne.

Pilot Movie – The Wedsworth-Townsend Act, Part Two

The second half picks up immediately after the surgery to replace the girl's arm. By the way, I forgot to mention in the other comments that at the boatyard, the guys start looking around for the missing limb (ugh!) and when Roy finds it he calls for Johnny to get the sterile sheet and saline solution, quick! My question is, why didn't they get those things out of the squad to take with them when they started the search? Time was of the essence, and every minute counted. Having to run to the squad for those things could take a full minute, at least. Anyway, we hear that the "re-attaching" surgery went better than expected and Brackett sat down for a civil cup of coffee with the guys before being called away to a "challenging" situation. Turns out that situation for which Dr. Early sought a second opinion involved yet another little kid (yes, another boy). And a French horn. And a bunny. So, just virtual minutes after Johnny refers to Brackett as a hard-a$$--er, I mean hard-nose--we see that same Dr. Brackett be very kind and gentle to a little boy.

4

We also see a woman stuck to her toilet seat. Yeah, business as usual at Rampart Emergency.

Dixie gets an idea all of a sudden and tells Brackett she's going to have a "wine and spaghetti get-together" for John Gage's birthday and wants Kel to be there. This is odd for a number of reasons. 1) in Part 1, my boyfriend Pete Malloy offered to buy Dixie a plate of spaghetti, for some odd reason; what if she'd wanted soup instead?? Anyway, this makes *two* mentions of spaghetti in the space of an hour. 2) I've never heard of a wine-and-spaghetti party before. Sounds messy, for one thing; much easier to go with cheese and crackers. 3) Dixie decided to have a party for Johnny's birthday... without checking to see if Johnny was available, much less get invites out to everyone else. I know, I know, it's just a TV show and I'm overthinking it, as usual. (By the way, I had the impression Johnny met Delores at the party; I didn't think she was his date.....??)

Speaking of the party, it was great to hear Dr. Early tickle the ivories and make up a little ditty about Dr. Brackett on the spot. (Supposedly.) Most of the rest of this scene is *not* great, including Roy's movie-wife, who is obviously not the same as his series-wife, even though we never see her. Anyway, I didn't like this version of her. Also, Johnny may have been a year older on his birthday, but here he acts like a surly eleven-year-old. Bad Johnny! And Brackett feels like he was being ganged-up on. He's still perfectly polite but he makes his exit only ten minutes after his entrance, and Dixie can't talk him into staying. This doesn't bode well for their personal relationship.

Next we see the guys and Dixie on the way to a car off the road in some remote area. I have no idea who called this in, and why there aren't any cops there. Chances are a deputy would have been closer than the paramedics and able to get there ahead of them. Anyway, a man has been thrown clear and a woman is still in the car, which is on its roof and teetering near the edge of a cliff. Dixie helps the guys extricate the woman, but before she can get out, the car rocks, and Dixie hits her head and gets knocked out. Roy and Johnny try to hold the car in place, each grabbing on as best they can, but then watch in horror as the car slips off the edge and turns into an only-on-TV fireball. But wait! As Roy said, the car must have pivoted around her as it fell. (What I want to know is, instead of trying to hold the car in place, why didn't the guys just grab Dixie's legs and pull her out? She was on the ground, for heaven's sake, all they had to do was yank her out from under.)

Anyway, now Dixie is victim #3, and Roy dials up Rampart "so they'll know we're going to [treat these patients]." After all, it's easier to ask forgiveness than permission. Brackett argues, Johnny says "hell," and the paramedics do their thing. (I do think it was childish--not to mention dangerous--for Johnny to turn off the link to base.) Also, when Roy asked Johnny how his victims were doing, Johnny says both are "in acute pain." How did he know that?? They were unconscious.

Boy, Dixie sure looks beautiful when she's in the hospital, doesn't she? Hair like a halo, attractive make-up... wishes I looked that good when I get all spiffed up for something. Kel isn't going to "blow the whistle" on the paramedics who went against his orders, and I admit I do like their little exchange at the end of the scene, when she says he's special and he replies "No, I'm not. But I'm glad you think so." I don't know why, but that just seems nice and sweet and, yes, sort of humble.

Then he goes and reams out those same paramedics that he's not blowing the whistle on. Roy stands his (their) ground and tells him they did their best in the time-critical circumstances. I know some may disagree, but I do believe that Brackett was just as correct as Roy was on most points: they did gamble by treating the patients, and if things had gone wrong, they would have set back emergency medicine by 10 years in LA County, and derailed the paramedic program for good. On the other hand, I hear Future Brackett telling Roy to "ask yourself if you're the best person available to give help, and if you are, pick up the ball and run with it." As it turns out, that's exactly what they did. (I still think Johnny was wrong to shut down the biophone, and this is where he should have acknowledged that, if not to Brackett, then at least to Roy.)

Unbeknownst to the paramedics (and even to Dixie) Brackett then goes to Sacramento to speak in front of the legislative committee in support of the Wedsworth-Townsend Act. I wonder if it was normal to have nobody else at the meeting; I guess it must be a closed committee? Anyway, it's another sad reflection of the times that Kel began his speech with "Gentlemen,......" Nope, no "ladies" in sight, except for the stenographer. But I thought his speech was eloquent and made the point about as well as it could be made.

Next comes the big mine rescue. My first question: WHY isn't there a nurse with them on this run? After having it beaten into our heads for over an hour, we know the paramedics aren't authorized to do anything more than give oxygen and apply bandages. They aren't there functioning as firefighters, they were brought in to assist with the wounded. And they carry in all their paramedic-y stuff, including the biophone and scope, etc. But I had to laugh at the melodramatic guy who said "It's terrible--terrible, dear God almighty!" Good heavens, how overblown and Webb-ish can you get?? And at the end, when they were getting ready to zap the victim with the bad heart.... was it just me or did it look like Johnny was taking his sweet time with the defibrillator? Time is of the essence, man, don't dawdle!!

One thing that kind of makes me frown is that everyone seems to change opinions at least once. Roy is all gung-ho about following the rules... until he isn't and he's ready to act on his own. Johnny's all het-up about having his hands tied and having to have a nurse do all the 'big' stuff... until he has to talk Roy down off the ledge and urge caution. Even Brackett, who all along has been opposed to the program, then grudgingly approving of it until something better comes along... now he's telling lies and tricking the guys into treating the patient. Man, I needed a scorecard to tell who was on which side of this issue at any given time.

We see that Johnny and Roy learn of Brackett's role in getting the bill passed, but Kel doesn't want to acknowledge that and says "la-la-la, I can't hear you" when they reference it. Roy calls Johnny "junior" and they get in the squad to go "back to the barn."

As the end credits roll, the viewer gets the feeling we may be seeing more of these two boys in the future.

Season One

1.1 Mascot

I haven't figured out why this episode is called Mascot... the subject in question can in no way be considered a mascot, especially for Station 51. But then, there are numerous times when the episode title doesn't seem to fit the show, so this isn't really a surprise.

In any case, it's rather jarring (to me, at least) that this ep has a 'cold' open—that is, it opens in the midst of action, with the squad racing to an accident scene. And John Gage's clipped, terse report "Squad 51, at scene" doesn't make me feel any more warm and fuzzy, either. (A Webb-esque holdover from the pilot movie, unfortunately.) In any case, the scene is apparently a single-car crash with a young woman behind the wheel. (Thank heaven there was no comment about "women drivers.")

The woman is slumped over the steering wheel and the bench seat is jammed forward, so of course it's sort of a production to get to her. But when they do.... I'm not gonna pretend we haven't all watched this show's later seasons (in other words, we're not E!-virgins) so I have to confess that I'm a little appalled at how they deal with her. Roy does take some care in leaning her head back on the headrest, but the way she writhes around and twists and turns in the seat is a little strange. And when they finally get things unjammed, I cringed as they pulled her out. No cervical collar, no backboard, nothing! Also, I had to laugh when Roy told Rampart that there was "very little" bleeding from her facial injuries. Really... we see more blood from these so-called minor cuts than we've seen from gunshot wounds and severed arteries. It's a good thing that Johnny already had the Ringer's IV bottle ready, even before Dr. Brackett asked for it. And I find it difficult to believe that "Bonnie" was so quiet and still during the whole time that the guys were working on her that nobody knew she was there. That just seems a little unrealistic to me.

In any case, Johnny goes with the young woman to Rampart. The good news is that Roy follows... *with* Bonnie. The bad news is that Johnny more or less promised Paula that he'd be sure that Bonnie is taken care of. And we all know what *that* means, don't we??

At the hospital, we see Johnny wandering around. He looks very young, very earnest, and... confused. Really, he looks like he'd never been to Rampart before, looking all around, doing double-takes when he sees an injured person, etc. And there did seem to be a number of people walking around with huge bandages on them. In any case, he finds Roy and then, well, it looks like Randy is acting, as in, reciting lines. I guess he hadn't gotten comfortable in the role or with his fellow actors yet, so that could be why he seems a little stiff in this episode. Also, I read that some of these first episodes were being filmed simultaneously with the pilot movie, so in fact these actors did not necessarily know each other that well, not to mention their own characters. Plus, I think they were still having to go strictly by the script. Later on the actors were given freedom to ad-lib and dialog flowed much more smoothly, but at this point, with you-know-who still somewhat in the picture, they probably toed the line pretty carefully.

Long story short, Johnny feels it's his responsibility to look after Bonnie for the duration, which makes things awkward at the station. Speaking of, this is the first time we see Captain Hammer. Dick Hammer—what a great name! Especially for a fire captain, which he was in real life. For the record, I always like Captain Hammer. He's no-nonsense and squared away, but not stiff. In fact, he's more natural with his lines than some actual actors. But I do like Hammer. By the way, I thought it was interesting when, in talking about Gage taking care of Bonnie, he said "If we get a bell, you make sure she's tied up." I don't think I've ever heard of it referred to as "a bell."

At Rampart, a woman brings her daughter to the Emergency Department—the daughter (a young married woman) is having trouble breathing. Now, maybe it's just me, and I've been watching this show too long, but it seems to me that it took two learned doctors and one very savvy nurse a really long time to come to the conclusion that the girl was simply hyperventilating. I guess they had to rule out other causes of her problem, and of course it's TV so they need to draw it out for dramatic purposes, I suppose. And then, what does Brackett do but have Dixie give the girl a 'tranquilizer.' This was the early '70s, after all... wasn't everyone popping tranquilizers like candy??

Does anyone else find it odd that the guys at the station play cards to determine who does dishes after a meal? On one hand, that does seem realistic, like something firefighters would do, but on the other hand, you'd think they'd have a better system in place. After all, the cooking is done on a rotation, so why wouldn't the clean-up be as well?

So Johnny's been trading shifts and working pretty much every day because of Bonnie. And sleeping in the camper parked behind the station. Did we ever discover whose VW van ("camper") that is? I'm pretty sure it's not Johnny's... if it was, he wouldn't have to stay at the station, he could park it in his own parking lot. Whoever it belongs to, it obviously stays parked behind the station all the time.

I always like the call to the party and the guy with chest pains. Kind of an odd time for a party (middle of the day), but you know those show-biz types, right?? But I thought that with the biophone, Rampart's side of the conversation is audible to anyone nearby through a speaker, so you'd think the stupid-jerk party guests would hear and realize it's really a doctor on the other end of the phone. By the way, in these early seasons, when the paramedics send a strip to the hospital, the machine at Rampart sounds just like one of the computers on the Enterprise from Star Trek. All that corny computerized screeching! But I do like the party rescue, and I'm glad the wife finally told all those "vultures" to get out. Always nice to see common sense rule the day, right?

We don't know what Johnny did with Bonnie when the squad gets called out on the hunting accident call… guess Hammer and Chet probably closed her up in one of the station closets, ha-ha. I'd put her in one of the showers with a bowl of food and the door firmly closed. Anyway, this is the first time we see our guys go up in a chopper.

This cliffside rescue is obviously (or so it seems to me) restaged elsewhere. When the guys are going from the chopper to the victim, the scene is very bright, in full sun. But when they get to the victim, suddenly the area is a lot darker, if not evening, then at least in deep shadow. All the scenes with the vic are like that, but when Johnny goes back up to the chopper, full sun again. So those victim scenes are filmed at either a different place or a different time, or, more likely, both. (I'm sure they didn't put our stars on that very real cliff ledge.) But I like that they experienced issues with line-of-sight to Rampart, impeding direct communications from the scene to the hospital. That's an issue that will be repeated again from time to time on the show, so it's interesting to establish that possibility.

Afterwards, we're at the station when Paula comes to retrieve Bonnie. The two are chatting somewhat shyly (like, I felt like I was watching a couple of 13-year-olds) and Johnny looks back meaningfully at Roy, as if to say "Get lost." But Roy can't go anywhere so he just shifts awkwardly in his chair, and then Johnny solves the problem by walking Paula out to her car.

At this point comes a very interesting exchange. Into the dayroom walks Chet, who passed John and Paula on their way out. Chet tells Roy, "Chicks really dig Gage," to which Roy replies, "That fatal charm of his is too much; sometimes he just can't turn it off." Now, on the face of it, that's all very well and good, but it seems as if the writers are setting us up for Johnny to be a chick magnet, someone who's so smooth that he has women clamoring for his attention.

And yet.... Well, we'll just have to watch the rest of the series to see how that plays out, right?? ;-)

Quick bits:

~ Nice to see Angelo DeMeo start his E! career in this episode (as an orderly). Same with Scott Gourlay.

~ In the dayroom, note the two tables are split.

~ There was a deputy/law enforcement officer in Rampart's emergency department. That actually makes total sense, and a lot of ERs do that, but as a rule we don't see it again here.

~ Who knew that John Gage is the long-john type? Not me. Maybe the Powers That Be didn't want to offend delicate 1972 sensibilities by showing us a guy in boxers. (If that's the case, they obviously get over it.)

~ When Johnny talked to Brackett at the cliff rescue, he identified as Rescue 51, but Brackett addressed them as Squad 51. At the heart-attack scene Johnny just said "This is 51."

~ ~ ~

About Mascot.... I had to kind of replay the call to the party, at which the man was having an apparent heart attack. The call came during the day, late morning or early afternoon or something, and there's a full-on party going on at this house, with people who I would think should probably be at some sort of job. (Wouldn't you think so?) They made reference to the man being an actor or something, but still.

Also, we didn't see the rest of Station 51 do anything in this episode, except in that first car accident where they got the dog, Bonnie. Otherwise it was the paramedic and doctor show, very light on firefighters, more's the pity. (Another thing that changed for the better as the show went on.)

1.2 Botulism

The Webb influence is still noticeable in this first season, with the awkward, unnatural-sounding dialogue. (Especially apparent after watching the later seasons, when the actors sound a lot more comfortable in their roles and dialogue is more natural.)

First off, it seems that Roy talks differently in these early episodes. Could be his inflection, or pitch, but I noticed it in the very first scene.

Speaking of the first scene, especially seeing it back-to-back with the final episode, All Night Long... we see Johnny reading, and also have discussion of him being on a "kick." It's almost like the two things are sort of book-ended, prominent in this early first-season episode, and again the last episode of the final season. Just an interesting coincidence, I thought.

In the footage of them driving to the first rescue, a different squad vehicle is used. Must have been from the pilot, as it's sort of early in the series for it to be stock footage, ya know?

At that rescue, why did Chet and Marco pull up the drug box and biophone, if Roy and Johnny didn't use it?? And the dialogue upon arrival at that rescue was awful. Same with the conversation with Nurse Wilma at Rampart. Referencing the pain the victim was in, Johnny says dramatically, "you'd think we'd get used to it," and Roy says "But you feel so helpless... we had the means." His delivery was *soooo* cheesy. I'm hoping Kevin was directed to deliver the line like that, rather than choosing to do it that way.

The time sequence at Rampart was a bit confusing: Brackett talks with the botulism guy's wife; he leaves office and runs into the press guys; Brackett says "no comment" and goes back into office; then suddenly Brackett arrives at the base station, as if he got there from inside his office. It was strange. (Maybe he has a secret passageway?)

Lightning round: I wonder who went back up the tower to get Johnny's turnout coat at that first rescue?? 'Cuz he left it there.... Brackett's wearing a POW bracelet. I remember I had one. ... The guy at the movie studio asked someone "would you give the wife a call." Really? "the wife"?? Bleah! ... What do people think of Early's hair? It wasn't the "Julius Caesar" 'do, but regular side part. I like it better this way. ... Dixie mentioned Lederle Labs, which I remember hearing about back in the day, for some reason (but *not* for botulism). ... Roy answered the 'red phone' at Rampart's base station, and it was for him! Maybe that was the procedure before they had an HT? ... Brackett looked quite young in these early days, but I have to say, I think Dixie looked better and better as the series went on. I also think Julie was much more attractive in the later '70s then she was in her publicity photos from 15 years earlier. (I like the 'softer' look.) ... This episode might have been the first reference to the Bird respirator. ... Also it gave us the first and (I think) last look at the Kennedy probe.   And the overshot, whatever that was. ... Station 51 is losing equipment early in the series, apparently. In that last rescue they lost a PortaPower and two prybars when that wall collapsed. ... I kind of like Capt. Hammer. He's really pretty decent in the role for not being an actor. I realize he left the show because it took up too much of his time, and I think the show did a smart thing by hiring an actor rather than another 'real' captain. ... Speaking of captains, the other captain on that final rescue had yellow tape on his helmet, likely to increase his visibility at night.

In this ep, I notice they wear the paramedic pins and name tags on their blue jackets, and they wear the jackets most of the time. But when they *don't* have the jackets on, the pins are on their uniform shirts. And I don't think they have two sets of pins, so what do they do, constantly switch them back and forth?

1.3 Cook's Tour

I confess that even the opening scene of this one kind of confused me. We see the squad running full-tilt with siren blaring along the city streets in the middle of the day. Cut to John and Roy inside the squad discussing who'll deliver the baby, and it looks like it's night out. Certainly no light coming in whatsoever. Maybe that's because it's such a tight camera shot and we don't see out the windows and thus no sunlight, but it certainly looks like it's dark. Then the squad pulls up to the house back in daylight (I've seen that same house in another episode of E! I believe, as well as an ep of Adam-12).

In the house, there is a convenient placement of chairs and other obstacles so as not to bruise delicate sensibilities by showing a woman in labor, never mind giving birth. Also, what about that horrendous hairy carpet they had in that room? I think the sole purpose of it was so we could see the woman dramatically clutching the 'fur' (shag) to artistically indicate the birthing process. (Hey ladies, newsflash... all you need is an ugly-*ss shag carpet, and childbirth is a breeze. Who knew!!!)

I thought it odd how R and J talked so openly to Rampart with the distressed mother and excitable father within easy earshot. Words like *stillborn, asphyxia* and *anoxia*... not to mention the phrase "we have a problem." **Umm, yikes.** I'd think those would be the kind of things they'd try *not* to say, so they don't upset the woman, y'know? Also, during the birth, shouldn't Johnny have been down by the woman's feet rather than kneeling next to her?? Last I checked, that's not where the baby comes out.

At Rampart, the wealthy woman whose son's hand was stuck in a vase was such a cliché of a 'society' woman: platinum upswept hair, large glasses, and wearing *fur* to the hospital, of all things. *eye-roll* Not to mention she looked more like the boy's grandmother than his mother.

Not once but twice in this episode we see Johnny and Roy do something that looks like unlocking the compartments of the squad. I think they were only pantomiming it (getting a key out, 'unlocking' it, putting key back in pocket), but the point is, they apparently kept the compartments locked at this point in the show. They did still leave the compartments wide open when they got their stuff out, but they took everything of value with them. Funny how much stuff--and how bulky it was-- they had to carry in the first season or so.

I heard Roy use his sexy-voice. also, this may be just me and I might truly be certifiable, but every time I hear the EKG strip at Rampart, I'm reminded of the sound of computers on the original Star Trek series.

Final rescue: why did they call for Engine 68 along with the squad? If they need an engine, I'd think they'd call the closest one, but the squad got to the scene well ahead of Engine 68. Also: I'm quite sure those were stunt guys. When we saw close-up of Johnny reaching the victim and he says "I hope you live to be a hundred" and hooked himself to the crane, I thought

I heard sort of an echo of that clanging sound; you don't hear echoes at 200 feet. And I'm not sure what the rope was for-- Johnny held one end and Roy held the other (it looked like), so I'm not sure what it was supposed to be doing. Lastly, when the guy fell, I saw that Johnny wasn't hooked onto anything. Roy was, but Johnny wasn't. Not very good form for a 'rescue man,' right? Also, this was Johnny's first "lost helmet." Take a drink!!

Lastly, is it just me or does it seem that either "Johnny" is awkwardly goofy in these early episodes, or that Randy is maybe over-acting a bit? Maybe it's just nerves about his first continuing role, but he seems to overdo it sometimes. Or maybe it's just the script, or what the director asked for? I don't know.

~ ~ ~

I think we've seen reference to the 'cook du jour' collecting money for groceries before (Botulism, maybe? or Mascot). But still you'd think Roy and Johnny would have told the clueless check-out girl to hang on to the bag they paid for and someone would pick it up. And yeah, that many groceries for 9 bucks? Wow, the good old days, huh? (I love TV-show grocery stores. They always have shelves that come up to shoulder or head height, and of course they're always neatly stocked.)

Don't you just love the prim and proper sensibilities of 1972? Thanks to very conveniently-placed chairs and boxes, we never see anything below the shoulders of the pregnant woman. And not a spot of blood or other child-birth goo. Yeah, cuz *that's* real!

I love Dixie's admonishment of "we don't run in this hospital-- ever." Funny, I've seen Brackett break that rule a time or two. And isn't it funny how Dr. Early gets to deal with all the kids?? (He of the potty-mouth in real life?)

Speaking of coffee, in the doctor's lounge or whatever they call that place, check out the ugly-butt lamp in the corner. World's ugliest piece of furniture!!

And this seemed to be a very Johnny-heavy episode. If anyone watched Mascot, the very first ep, at the very end it seems as if the show is setting Johnny up as the charming ladies' man. Roy and Chet talk about how all the chicks seem to 'dig' him and "he can't turn off the charm," etc. Oddly, that's not how things shape up later in the series, when Gage seems to strike out a lot more often than he gets to first base. Ah well, at least the writers are going to quietly drop the Dixie-and-Brackett relationship. That just seemed awkward all the way around.

You mention no hospital security... what I wonder about is the no-fee policy. Patients leave the treatment rooms and just walk out the door. No forms to sign, no fees to pay--nothing! How did Rampart stay in business?? And speaking of Rampart, it occurred to me today... Dixie says she'll get treatment room 2 or something ready for 51's patient, and their ETA is 20 minutes. What if they get flooded with other emergencies in the meantime? "I'm sorry, we can't treat your profusely-bleeding stab wound, we're all full up and we don't have room for you. We have a hyperventilating man with a nail in his toe coming in anytime now."

~ ~ ~

Just watching Cook's Tour again--for no valid reason-- and in one rescue, the guys respond to a man who was electrocuted while fixing his washing machine (or dryer, or something). First of all, they identify him as being "40" years old. If he's forty, then I'm 30. (And I'm not 30.) Anyway, when they first get to him, Johnny puts his hand on the guy's neck and says "BP is off the page" (which I assumed means high). A few minutes later, after starting an IV and getting ready to transport, Johnny picks up the paper where Roy had jotted down vitals and tells

Rampart "blood pressure is very low, 60 over 20." Either they didn't pay attention to their own script, or that D5W took effect real quick. To be fair, when Johnny said the BP was 'off the page,' I suppose he *could* have meant low. But my initial reaction was that he meant it was very high.

* * *

Also in this episode, we actually see Johnny unlock the compartment on the squad. I'm not sure we've ever seen them do that before. (Have we???) Of course, once he takes the trouble of unlocking it and getting the stuff they need, what do they do then but walk away.... and leave the compartments wide open. Yeah, they leave the compartment doors open all the time, I've noticed, no matter where they are. Of course, they usually have their hands so full of stuff, I don't see how they'd have a spare hand to close them, much less lock 'em.

1.4 Brushfire

Okay, the first time we see Station 51 at a brushfire. Not to be confused with that other brushfire episode we'll see later on in the series. By the way, were we all impressed with the real fire footage used in this episode? Unfortunately I'm sure there's no lack of it. Anyway, I was caught off guard by the fact that, at the station, we could hear the radio broadcast of one of the engines or brush units calling *in* to LA dispatch. Usually we can't hear those incoming calls, just the dispatch's side. Anyway, random thoughts in no particular order:

Re the little old ladies... their house was the infamous house from Psycho. I read an article that the house has been used numerous times for TV or movies, sometimes being relocated from one place to another. The article mentioned this episode of E! as one of the shows/movies that house has been seen in.

Speaking of the old lady, and her 'wild ride' to the hospital, I can't believe they didn't use a bungie cord or even a rope to secure the stokes on the back of the squad. One big bump and she would've gone sailing over that little railing.

I noticed Station 51's captain has been acknowledging calls with "Station 51, 10-4." I'll try to listen to when he starts saying KMG-365.

The baby delivery in this episode is one of my favorite scenes, for some reason. Again, we don't 'see' anything, but it's funny (and clever) how Johnny 'narrates' what's happening while on the biophone to Rampart. And by the way, on the subject of delivering babies, I wonder if there were any conversations at the time (1972) about writing a scene with an unmarried young man like Johnny delivering a baby as he did in an earlier episode. I know at one time unmarried female nurses were not allowed to attend to male patients, for propriety's sake, but I guess that convention and concern for delicate sensibilities didn't apply to unmarried men attending to ladies--and their 'lady parts.'

And by the way, I don't believe I've ever heard that "pressing down on the ribs" of a pregnant woman can help facilitate childbirth. Yeah, that's good to know!!

Dialogue is still pretty stilted sometimes. I counted two instances of people responding to comments with "You know it." Not sure when (if ever) I've heard someone say that... today's translation would be "I know, right?" But the worst, most awkward is the dialogue on the biophone to Rampart. I know they don't have all day and have to relay information quickly, but in these early episodes they're awfully stingy with their vocabulary... you'd think they have to pay by the word!

"Injured fireman, beneath a tree. Leg pinned. Crimped pretty good. Arterial bleeding." Almost sounds like he's dictating a telegram. "Leg pinned-stop. Arterial bleeding-stop." Can't wait until the actors are free to ad-lib and take control over their characters!

* * *

Actually, about the delicate act of delivering a baby and the glimpsing of 'lady parts' during childbirth, my curiosity was about the woman's sensibilities as much as the unmarried man's. Theoretically, back in these ancient days of the early '70s, nobody saw a woman's nether-regions except her doctor and her husband (and maybe not even her husband... if they kept the lights off in the bedroom *wink*). And her doctor seeing her was okay because he (most likely a he) was a well-educated doctor, revered and exalted as they were back in the day. Next down on the list of 'men who can see the bikini area' would be medically trained married men... and the 'married' part could be important because at least nothing he saw would shock him or be something he hadn't encountered before. But an unmarried young man? A man who (again, theoretically) had never seen a woman 'down there' before?? Why, the woman could feel violated, as if a voyeur, a mere nobody, had peeked into her undies. And as for the young man, what he sees 'down there' could unleash some primal animal urges in him and cause him to go wild. (Ha-ha, I really should write this stuff down. Either that or I should get a life.)

~ ~ ~

This one was directed by Hollingsworth Morse, who not only directed quite a bit for Adam-12, but also directed a number of episodes of the infamous Operation Petticoat (a sitcom in which Randy had a role... which nobody has seen but everyone is curious about, am I right?). Anyway this is the only E! ep directed by Morse, surprisingly.

When the guys are all looking at the map for the location of the brush fire, which is in a newly-developed area, Captain Hammer says "In that area the streets are laid out by goats." Huh?? Is that a saying I never heard of before??

Then, when they leave to go to the brush fire, they turn *right* out of the station. I have no idea where Station 51 (127) is in relation to anything else in LA County (although I know it's in Carson), but I always assumed that going right would take them 'toward town' and turning left is out toward the boonies.

Did you see where the TV was in the doctor's lounge? Not next to the door, as usual. Also, was it just me or did Roy sound a little like he had a cold? On the plus side, we did get to hear more of his sexy-voice.

I think we talked about this before, but again, I didn't see Johnny tie down the stokes with little old Miss Winifred on there. She could've blown away in a breeze.

Not sure when this was filmed, but it looked cold. In that scene when Johnny brought Roy some coffee (as they leaned on the hood of the hood of the squad), you could see their breath.

The Webb Effect, or just preferred paramedic protocol? Referring to the clipped tones of communication on the biophone. Almost never complete sentence. Like this. Or this: "Fireman trapped. Arterial bleeding. Tourniquet has been applied." (Verdict: don't like it. Glad it went away.)

When Roy volunteers to respond to the pregnant woman call, he honks the horn to get Johnny's attention, and Johnny just jumps right in the squad and they drive away. He looked like an eager puppy happy to go for a ride (wonder if he stuck his head out the window like a puppy). I suppose Johnny might have heard the announcement, but he didn't even ask Roy where they were going.

Was it just me or did Roy seem almost a little creepy with that pregnant woman? *WE* know he's a good guy and wouldn't hurt a fly, but some of his comments could be construed differently under other circumstances. "Everything's under control... Are you here alone?... We're gonna take care of you." Hmm, maybe Roy has a doll named Chucky...??

How long did that pregnant-woman call take, anyway? It was full dark when they were at her house, but full daylight when they left the hospital after dropping her off.

Wally Cleaver is a looter? June and Ward would be sooo disappointed. And his hair had grown out quite a bit, too, since he'd been carjacked on Adam-12. What I was wondering though, was if it was his *shoulder* that was hurt, why was he still lying down? A knee or ankle injury I could understand leaving him stuck on the ground. But a shoulder? He should have been up and been able to hide or toss the 'loot' by the time the squad got there.

This too was mentioned before, but still... it bothers me that Roy and Johnny just tied the dog to the phone booth and were going to leave. They didn't even know if the boy was still at Rampart, much less when he'd be leaving; they couldn't possibly have known he was on his way out the door (from an oddly-located treatment room, no less).

1.5 Dealer's Wlld

I like this episode. Quite a bit, actually. I like all the rescues, and Johnny's "kick of the week" didn't bother me. (Not sure why... maybe because he was upbeat about coming up with a new game, and wasn't irritable and scowling at anyone.)

~ Dispatcher Sam signed off on a call as "LA clear, KMG-941." We may hear that once or twice in the first season, but I don't think any more than that.

~ Love the plane rescue! And how lucky that Roy has a little flying experience. What would they have done if he hadn't, I wonder?? Also, I thought that airport attendant looked a little (in a very general way) like Kent McCord. Maybe it was his less-attractive cousin.

~ Speaking of that rescue (and how great Roy/Kevin looked while talking to the young boy), was it just me or did the scene of the airport and landscape, from the air, not match what we saw from the ground?? From the air it looked all flat and empty, but from the ground the 'airport' looked like a glorified parking lot.

~ Once they got the plane pilot on the ground and to Rampart, it was cute to see Roy sit the boy down in the reception area and hand him a magazine. Also, I think *this* boy, Frankie, would have been a good one for Roy to take home with him for a night or two. Much better than the terror (Eddie) he ends up with in season 5. Frankie would've appreciated Roy and his family.

~ Brackett was wearing the same shirt in this ep that he wore in. Speaking of Brackett's clothes.... I think my brain had a mini-stroke when trying to take in the outfit he wore to Dixie's apartment (the first time). Pants and shirt had different striped patterns, and his tie had yet a third pattern. (I tried to get a photo but there wasn't a good angle that showed the full effect.) And then, to add insult to injury, he wore a similar (but different?) pair of striped pants the next day, with yet a different-patterned shirt. Add Dixie's dress into the mix.... yikes, my eyes still haven't adjusted.

~ The overturned tanker at the friendly neighborhood (and ubiquitous) oil refinery.... did I miss something? I didn't see any spilled gasoline. But I'll take their word for it, I guess. On the plus side, Johnny got to use the little tool they wear on their bunker coats (spanner wrench?). I always think that's so cool that they wear that around.

~ I thought it odd that Johnny gave Rampart the victim's name and address. Not sure how that's relevant in the least, but then, I don't write for the show.

~ Also odd that Brackett requested an EKG and immediately a strip came in. Last we saw, the paramedics hadn't even patched him in... they were lucky they had his BP by that point.

~ I wonder what those albums were at Dixie's place? Maybe some Julie London jazz? Bobby Troup piano tunes??

~ Lastly, please tell me I'm not the only one who wonders what happened to the elevator at Rampart? Apparently the hospital hasn't installed elevators yet, and the door at the end of the hallway (near the base station) is still a utility treatment room. But I do a double-take every time I see anything other than elevator doors there.

~ ~ ~

Okay, so here goes.

~ I've noticed a couple times in season 1 the two tables in the kitchen/rec room have been separated... usually some books/notebooks on one of them. And an ash-tray. Glad they don't show anyone smoking! Speaking of the books, we often see the guys reading manuals or other type of books... wish they'd mention if they're taking extra classes or something.

~ You'd think they'd have a better way to decide who does dishes. As in, whoever doesn't cook, cleans up. The cook shouldn't have to do dishes as well.

~ I heard Captain Hammer say KMG-365. Yay. But only once, and not the next time. Boo.

~ Brackett's wacky wardrobe!! Two different types of stripes (shirt, pants) and a tie with yet another type of design/pattern. When he took his coat off at her apartment, Dixie said "You do look tired." I expected her to say "You do look tired--you must've been half asleep when you got dressed."

~ At the tanker truck site, the foam totally obscured and got all over the box from the porta-power. I wonder if they even remembered to get the porta-power back.

~ Johnny got to drive to a call!! Woo-hoo!!

~ A "subarachnoid blowout," huh? Sounds like it's just up Brackett's alley— spiders on the brain!

This was kind of a dark episode, especially for this show. For one thing, they mentioned someone slashing their wrists. There have been attempted suicides on this show before (or, perhaps I should say there will be, later), but usually it's just pills or maybe carbon-monoxide (??). But slashing wrists... that's kinda dark. And they kinda almost showed some blood too, with the deputies holding his arms. Plus, the boy's pilot father died, leaving him an orphan. That's two bad things in one episode.

Also, it seems as if the dialogue is starting to improve already. Not as stilted and Webbish. Or maybe it's just this one episode... we'll see. Oh, and I loved "Roy to the Rescue" with the plane thing. He's generally laid-back and easygoing, but I love it when he takes charge.

~ ~ ~

Again, I know it was the early '70s when this show began, and I shouldn't judge wardrobes by today's standards. But I have to say it's so weird (to me, at least) to see these guys 'dressing up' to go to work. I mean, they get to the station and they change into a uniform, so it's not like anybody (i.e., the public) sees them in their 'soft' clothes. When they get off work at 8:00 in the morning they're probably going to just go straight home, so why not be a little more casual? (I was young enough that I didn't pay attention to these things, but I wonder when adults started wearing t-shirts [nice, presentable ones, I mean] out in public.)

And yeah, Dixie's dress was pretty wild... like something you'd see on Laugh-In.

By the way, I don't think I've ever heard that saying about "grass won't grow on a playground." Or if I did, it was so long ago that I don't remember.

Edit: going back to the episode.... In the airstrip scene, after all that Roy did to talk the boy down in the plane, get the kid to put oxygen on his dad, treat the dad once the plane landed, walk the kid into the hospital, etc. ... after all that, Brackett is the one the boy hugs. Go figure!!

*   *   *

You haven't seen Captain Hammer yet?? Better catch him quick before he's gone.

And yeah, that 'dressing up' to go to work thing does puzzle me. You go directly to work, where you're going to change into a uniform and nobody will see you in your own clothes, and on top of that, you get off work at 8:00 a.m. If you got off work at 5pm or 8pm, I could see that you might want to stop by a friend's house, or meet friends for a drink (or a date), but at 8 in the morning?? Maybe there's some clause or requirement that you dress nicely on your way to/from work, as whether on duty or not you're a 'representative' of the county or hospital or whatever entity you work for. Yes? No? Just spit-balling here, but it always does seem odd. (I've noticed the same issue on Adam-12 as well, so it's not just Emergency that has me wondering this.)

> I swear I've seen Roy come out and button his uniform shirt with nothing on underneath. And occasionally you see Johnny in the white tank tops commonly referred to as "wife beaters" (I hate that term), although I can't remember if that was on or off duty, when he's been changing at the lockers.

You *have* seen Roy put on his uniform shirt without a t-shirt underneath. We'll see it from time to time in the series. (And I'm not complaining, mind you.) And you're also correct about Johnny wearing a 'wife-beater' (I hate that term too.) but yes, I believe (?) it's usually when he's changing clothes *from* his street clothes, as in, that's Johnny's shirt and not part of the uniform.

I had never really heard that native Americans have 'smooth skin' (i.e., no body hair) until recent conversations about Johnny and Roy in the locker room. (Is it weird that that's an actual conversation topic??) I tend to prefer a little bit of frontal fur... not too much, but some... just a little to prove that Y chromosome. As I've said before, it gives a girl something to hold onto.

1.6 Nurse's Wild

I won't rehash the sterile cleanliness of the gunshot wound victim again. Or the nice, dressy Sunday-go-to-robbing shirt he's wearing. Speaking of clothes, someone made the observation that in Season 1 the paramedics are wearing their blue jackets a lot. And yeah, they really are. A *lot*. I wonder why, especially when most of the other FFs aren't.

~ Roy did a little "executive decision" action in disagreeing with Rampart on countershocking the store owner. Take charge, Roy! Also, when he arrived at the hospital, we see Roy walking in the Emergency entrance, but he obviously didn't park next to the ambulance. I thought that was interesting. Speaking of Roy taking charge, I always love his handling of the 'guard dog' in this episode. Interestingly, there's an Adam-12 episode in which Malloy also gets creative in dealing with a large guard dog. Gotta love the symmetry!

~ This was an episode with a number of familiar faces. Or at least, they will *become* familiar as the series goes on. **The robber,** Clive, was played by Kip Niven, who appeared 2 other times on this show (once as the trainee who had the persistent cough). **The hallucinating man** was a character actor who played one of the old coots--one thumped the other on the chest real hard, remember? (And he's also immortalized in the out-take in the blooper reel with Bobby Troup.) **The deputy,** who's unnamed in this episode, later goes on to be referred to as Vince (which is handy because that's the actor's name). And **the encyclopedia salesman** who told them about the dog in the house is also a repeat guest-star, as a floor-cleaner and also as the "professional patient."

~ Had to laugh at Roy's comment to Marco. Marco asked the "doctors" about an echo he kept hearing in his head, and Roy said "What do you expect from a big empty space, bells?" Ha! (And yes, I'm still loving the sexy-voice on him.)

~ Sam finishes another call-out with "LA clear, KMG-941."

~ This time we hear Dr. Morton swear ("d--- it"). And how cool, his patient was the guy who plays the lead in Jesus Christ, Superstar. (Ha, just kidding about that.) I have to say, that patient got the quickest lab results in history. Less than a minute after Morton draws the blood, they get the call about the test results.

~ The last call-out to the "chemical plant" was at the corner of Manson and 10th Street. I have to cringe every time I hear the name Manson. As of this episode it had only been a little over a year since the Manson trial. I'd think they could have used some other street name rather than put that one in everyone's mind again. Oh, and at this rescue, Roy and Johnny weren't wearing gloves (again!) when lowering the victim down with the ropes. Bet they had some pretty good callouses on their hands from this show!

* * *

Yeah, the "women's vanity" and "men's blindness" thing was a good interplay between Dixie and Brackett. Too bad it didn't get delved into further. Dixie could've pointed out that, in addition to being blind, men can be vain too. But I'm glad the "dating" thing between these two was dropped. Just a distraction.

* * *

I totally agree about Morton taking his criticism well. And twice, too, as you mention. It was a good little detail to see him taking his lumps like a man and apologizing to the guy. And while we didn't see him apologize to the nurse, I'm sure he did. As for Brackett, maybe he learned his lesson about bedside manner just from listening to Dixie, and that's what made the lightbulb in his head go off and he was nice to Grace, the young woman who took the diet pills. (By the way, I've noticed that 'back in the day,' it wasn't called 'dieting,' but instead 'reducing.' In this episode, and in at least one other one that I recall--involving Dr. Early--it's referred to as reducing. Just semantics, I guess.)

Also by the way, here's an odd bit about Nurse Bart: she's listed in the credits as Ellen Bart, but her name tag clearly shows her name to be Barnett.

~ ~ ~

Random thoughts about Nurse's Wild....

~ Gunshot wound to abdomen, and Johnny says "slight blood loss visible." WTF, how does that work? We've seen more blood from a car crash victim hitting her head on the steering wheel (in Mascot) than we did for a gunshot. Also, aren't these crooks nicely dressed? Just like firefighters, no jeans allowed, apparently. (Among Adam-12 fans it's kind of an in-joke that crooks always wear slacks and windbreakers.)

~ This episode featured hospital pages for both Dr. Jose Estrada, and "Stat Ident."

~ Remember the brushfire episode when Johnny tied up the lost-but-then-found dog to the phone booth outside the emergency entrance*? Today that same area outside Rampart didn't have phone booths; they were covered up by some plasterboard or something. But you could see where they'd been.

~ Anyone have a clue why Johnny asked Roy about Indian Guides? He had a date with Nurse Ellen for Friday, and then he suddenly said "Friday night? Isn't that when you take your kid to Indian Guides?" What does that have to do with Johnny's date? Does he need Roy to chaperone his dates? And speaking of the nurse, Johnny calls her a 'wild chick,' and says she has funny ideas and peculiar attitudes. Does that mean he feels confident about getting lucky?? That would be my bet.

~ It's been mentioned that this is the ep in which Johnny recites the rundown on all the Rampart nurses: who's married, who's the "right age" and "right weight." I have to grit my teeth and close my ears during that speech, reminding myself that it was the unenlightened early '70s. Not to mention the storyline at Rampart with girl who took the diuretics for 'reducing' so she could get a date.

~ Lastly, it's funny to watch this show with closed captioning from Netflix. The closed-captioning states that in the background the dispatcher says that "Italian 7 is responding." (Supposed to be *Battalion* 7.)

* About that phone booth thing... I can't believe Johnny just tied the dog to the booth and was going to drive away. What if the kid left by another door (it is the emergency entrance, after all). What if he'd had to stay at the hospital another day? What if someone else had taken the dog, or it had gotten loose again?? Those things bother me. (Yeah, I'm weird like that.)

*   *   *

About the table at the station... it's actually two separate tables, each about three feet wide, that are normally pushed together. Here in the first season, we're seeing them separated quite a bit, but both in the same rec/kitchen room. But still, there are two of them. In later seasons, they're almost always pushed together to make one big table.

Good thought about the dog, that maybe Roy and John called to let Dixie know. I hadn't thought of that. To me it looked like they tied up the mutt, walked away, and would have left if Dixie and the kid hadn't come out so soon. If they expected her, why wouldn't they just hold the leash and wait. Ah well, it's small potatoes (as my boss used to say).

But that comment about the Indian Guides.... that's the kind of thing that bothers me. Makes me wonder if there was a scene or other dialogue somewhere that was cut in editing, because it was very deliberately mentioned (i.e., not just background conversation). The only other thing I can think of is that on one hand, the topic is the girl's "wild attitudes and peculiar ideas" and Roy says "that's quite a combination, her peculiar attitudes and your one-track mind." On the other hand, Johnny points out that Roy will be taking his kid to Indian Guides. Maybe they're pointing out the contrast in how to spend a Friday night-- one has a date with a "wild chick," and the other will be at a family-friendly kiddie event. Ah well, guess we'll never know. (Cue the bizarre fan-fic sub-plot.)

1.7 Publicity Hound

So, there's an episode about a "great paramedic" who gets all the press and attention, and John Gage gets jealous, huh? Gee, that sounds familiar. Except that the paramedic isn't Craig Brice, it's Tom Wheeler. Guess the writers began recycling storylines later in the series. (And actors too... yesterday's fireman Conway is today's paramedic Wheeler.)

So, let's get on with the minutiae....

~ In the first scene Johnny mentioned a cracking tower, so of course I had to look it up: it's a tower used at a petroleum refinery to help, well, refine petroleum. (I didn't grow up in an oil state, so if I ever knew what a cracking tower was, I'd long since forgotten it.)

~ The rescue on the boat: I think it's a cool rescue, and they had to get creative to get the victim down. I do have to wonder though, about jurisdiction. Wouldn't the Coast Guard be the first call rather than LACoFD? Or maybe they weren't far enough out in the water?

~ I still call bogus on the John Gage seasickness thing. He didn't look seasick at all, during the boat ride out to the schooner or on the mast of the schooner. Maybe it was sympathy seasickness?? See a pretty girl barf and then *you* go barf.

~ The horse 'rescue': Johnny, Johnny, you just try too hard with the ladies, and all it gets you is in a ditch looking at the business end of a horse. And speaking of the ditch and the horse, he came pretty darn close to hitting that horse with the shovel handle. Not cool, Gage, not cool at all. (Although I think it was funny/mean that Roy made Johnny do all the work.)

~ So this is the beginning of the undeniable DeSoto magnetism. Try as he might (again: too hard), Johnny stands on the sideline and watches women flock to Roy. Roy who supposedly has no charisma. Ha!

~ Speaking of Roy, did anyone see him lose his pen (or something) at the construction site? He was on that ladder looking into the hole for the little girl, and something fell out of either his pants pocket or his shirt pocket.

~ ~ ~

Re the boat rescue, was anyone else channeling the old pirate movies of yore? The episode could have been called "Yo-ho-ho and a bottle of Ringer's." First off, why is it called a bosun's chair, when it's not really a chair but more of a harness? And while the other day, Johnny ran up the pipes in that factory rescue while Roy was more hesitant, today Roy looked like he was born to sail, while Johnny was the one who was cautious. Not sure why Johnny was suddenly (supposedly) sea-sick, though, he didn't really show any sign of being nauseous or even queasy. But as soon as the girl in the bikini top ran by, off goes Johnny to christen the ocean. (While they all stood around chatting just seconds after saying how critical the time factor was for their victim.)

Once again Brackett and Early did surgery in the ED, even though there's an entire room and staff dedicated for *just* that purpose. And in that scene after surgery, with the two doctors talking in the break-room, Brackett pours himself a cup of coffee, giving us a clear view of his P.O.W. bracelet. (Remember those?? I had one when I was young!) And I can't believe that Mr. Dumont guy... why was he (or they) discussing his son's condition in front of other people? Brackett should have insisted on privacy before even talking about it.

So we see Dr. Morton as an intern. Brackett said Early should bring his students (interns) on the rounds, and voila, there's Morton.

With the horse 'rescue,' once again, or perhaps I should say, for the first time in the series, we see the low-key DeSoto charm get better results than the Overeager Gage Method. Kind of upends the scene in the first episode, Mascot, when it looked like the writers were setting Johnny up as someone who gets all the female attention.

Good point about the little girl not being injured and suffering nothing more than being scared and dirty. What I wondered about that rescue was why, with a full professional construction crew and all that equipment, it was the *paramedics* who had to dig the final tunnel to reach the girl. It's not like, even if she had been injured or something, they could have done anything for her in that 15-foot hole in the ground. I think that falls under what has been called the "cheesy TV manipulation" category. After all, how exciting would a show about paramedics be if they didn't do all the rescues?

The dialog in this ep was a little more Webb-ish than we'd seen recently. Interestingly, it seems that for the 7 episodes we've seen so far, there have been six writers. Publicity Hound was written by the same guy who did Botulism, but the other five eps have all been written by different people.

*   *   *

I noticed how everyone in the station basically had the same haircut. Tim Donnelly supposedly grew his mustache to be more recognizable, which certainly worked. As their hair styles and facial hair started to vary, they all looked so much alike, even having their hair parted on the same side.

I've noticed that too.... during this first season, Roy's the only one with light hair. But they all do have the same exact cut, complete with right-side part. Marco and Chet? interchangeable, especially from more than 10 feet away (and they're the same size). So yeah, they all have the same 'do in this first season or so. And when they have their helmets on.... good luck telling who's who!

1.8 Weird Wednesday

Yes, this *was* kind of a weird episode... and not really notable, imho. For one thing, we barely get to see the "other" guys of Station 51; we see them at the station, and very marginally at the parachute rescue.

Which reminds me... what did that county deputy mean by "Lady parachutist"?? Should we call him a "man cop"? Is Brackett a "dude doctor"? That deputy called her a 'lady parachutist' with the same tone of voice people used to harrumph and say 'women drivers.'

Speaking of the woman in the tree, she tells Johnny (referring to her chute) "pull the cover down and squeeze." I want to know why she couldn't do that? In the words of every 12-year-old everywhere, "your arms aren't broke."

After the deal with the guy in the freezer, John and Roy were talking in the squad, referring to what they do "in the Himalayas," and talked about "zapping yourself in and out at any time." I presume they were talking about meditation, or hibernation, or trances or something? There wasn't much context offered to us viewers, except what they'd been told about the kid being able to slow his breathing.

In this episode it seems that time itself is affected by weirdness, too. After the freezer rescue, as they pulled into the station, it looked like evening... lights were clearly on on the outside of the station. Yet, they're in the station no more than 2 minutes before being called out again, and as they're driving it looks like late afternoon (based on shadows). But when they're treating the girl on the golf course, the sun is obviously higher in the sky. So time must have been going backward on them. (Time of call was 3:33. Supposedly.) Oh, and btw, Roy uses his sexy-voice on that call.

I noticed they used the plastic IV bags in this one (with snake-bite girl), but the hospital still used the glass bottles. Personally I don't know how the paramedics could have stored those huge, bulky bottles. Also, this call is good preparation for Johnny in case some day *he* gets bitten. Lastly, I wonder what book Roy was reading at the very end, before their last call-out. Almost looked like those old-fashioned Harlequin books, but obviously it wasn't. I hope.

* * *

Yeah, that scene with the hooker. You'll notice that nothing was ever actually *said*... all we saw was some eye-rolling and all we heard was gum-snapping (uber annoying!!). But I wonder what the average 12-year-old in 1972 thought she was, or what the two of them were doing? Since she never said *anything* there wasn't even a double-entendre, giving some people one interpretation while others might get a different one. There was just.... no explanation at all. The words "hotel" or "bar" or "picked up" weren't used. She didn't even call him John (instead, it was Freddie). I bet there were a lot of *adults* back in '72 who never got what was going on in that scene. (And maybe some still don't.)

As for the snakebite victim's pantyhose... I never cared for the nude color, I always liked tan. The hit on my sensibilities comes from wearing pantyhose while playing golf.

Yeah, I just wish there had been more clarification on that little scene about the measured breathing. Although from the things they said, it almost sounded as if they were referring to some sort of trance, as Johnny said something about "it's probably not that hard to get yourself into it," and Roy replies with "yeah, but I wonder how you get yourself out of it." (Total paraphrasing, but that is the gist.)

You mention the ambulance drivers and their white clothes. Why is it that people whose jobs might get them dirty or stained wear white?? Doctors, nurses, ambulance drivers... even house painters. I've always wondered why painters are portrayed as wearing white when they have the big likelihood of getting 'stuff' on them??

~ ~ ~

Johnny never does explain why, even at the start of the day (shift) he thought it was going to be a strange day. This would have been a good episode for those weird calls from dispatch (Samoan fire-dancer, child stuck on elephant, etc.).

In any case, thanks to the first call, we got to see Johnny's gymnastic leap off the squad. Always fun to watch!

First call is to the "lady parachutist." Would the deputy have called it a "guy parachutist" if he'd been male?? And how annoying is that woman, anyway?? I can't stand when people keep repeating their statements/comments/questions and either don't wait for an answer, or don't bother listening to it when it comes.

Speaking of that scene, where did those onlookers and bystanders come from? It's not like this happened in a commercial area, or even a residential area. The woman landed in a tree in the middle of nowhere, and yet there are six-eight people standing around watching. And it's not like parachutists make a lot of noise to attract people. *eye-roll*

Had to laugh when Johnny used the saw and then came away with a small branch barely an inch in diameter. That made the woman feel so good she climbs all over Roy--literally--as she gets down the ladder.

Later, when the squad arrives at the scene with William Katt and his father, listen to Sam's dispatch to Squad 209; I could swear he says "Haystack in the dairy." Whatever that means. (Maybe Squad 209 is having a Weird Wednesday, too.) Also, William Katt needs to learn how to dress properly. When you're going jogging you should never wear A) fugly shorts like those, or B) shorts that have belt loops on them. Yikes!!

I don't know about anyone else, but I cringe whenever I see one of those old station-wagon style ambulances. They look like hearses.

Haven't we seen the persistent hiccup problem before? Or rather, we will. Dr. Early gets hiccups at some point, I believe, and a little kid has the answer on how to get rid of them. And I love when Brackett says that while he still had the hiccups, the patient is of no use to anyone except "as a metronome." Too funny, doc! (When I was a kid, I used to get hiccups almost every time I ate mashed potatoes. True story!)

Is it me or is it odd that the woman was golfing by herself? I know people do golf solo sometimes, but usually the point of golf is to hang out with 2 or 3 friends. And drink; can't forget the drinking. But we do get to hear the sexy-voice again.

(Which makes me think of "Dr. Sexy, M.D." If you know what that's from.... "awesome!")

So this episode actually addresses the world's oldest profession with the foreign guy who's brought to the hospital in the cab. The show goes out of its way to NOT say what he was doing, or who the girl was who brought him in. Although I have to say, she was the most "girl next door"-looking hooker I've ever seen, y'know? But it was funny when the man found someone he could talk to and she interpreted for the man, and when asked to find out "where he hurts," the nurse said "he can't tell me." Does that mean he doesn't know, or that he doesn't want to tell the pretty nurse about some 'man-pain' he's having? Has it been longer than four hours, perhaps???

Johnny hurt his knee going down to see the plastered drunk driver. Is this Johnny's first-ever owie??

Lastly, I like when Dr. Early said there's only one cure for the "weird" day: "Eventually it'll be tomorrow." Not soon enough for Johnny, doc! Also, that line reminded me of the title of an episode of Route 66, "Somehow It Gets to be Tomorrow." (That's kind of a long and awkward title for an episode, but Route 66 has some doozies for titles) Anyway, it all sort of ties in because Bobby Troup wrote a famous song about route 66... even though ironically it was *not* the theme for the TV show.

* * *

The whole foreign-speaking sailor story was just odd. Didn't it finally turn out that his wrist hurt? That's a far cry from a heart attack. How the heck did he hurt it and why wouldn't he be able to tell the nurse? Oh well, it is Weird Wednesday after all.

Yeah, it was odd, wasn't it?? The man did tell the nurse his wrist hurt, but then he talked some more and hung his head and she said "he can't tell me." Kinda makes you wonder what *else* he hurt, doesn't it??

>   Interesting that John knew how to hotwire the squad after
>   Roy broke off the ignition key.

Yeah, I wonder where Johnny learned how to do that, right?? And he'd have to do it for the whole shift until they could get the end of the key out. How do you do that, anyway? Thin tweezers?? A magnet??? I assume they have extra keys available.

As for the mirror, you never see the mirror when looking *into* the squad, because there's no need for one. With the box style of the truck, there's nothing to look at in a rear-view mirror. But when filmed looking *out of* the squad, they obviously use a different truck, one that has room for a cameraman behind the seat. It's a continuity error that they don't fix the discrepancy. Hmm, offhand I don't recall a scene looking out of the squad in this one. I've seen it before, but didn't catch it in this one. Good eye!

1.9 Dilemma

Yeah, Johnny cooked his own goose in this one, didn't he? And he deserved it. Hurray for Roy and his (usual) common sense. I agree that whole "calling a girl a do" thing is painful to hear, I think a similar conversation comes up in another episode along the way. Although in this one Roy says Cynthia is "what *you* would call a dog," so he's distancing himself from that characterization while acknowledging that's what Johnny would say.

About the student nurse Walters... I wrote a whole post on it somewhere on this board and I think I titled it "Dixie blew it," because in my opinion, she really did. It's her job to see that the ED runs smoothly, and first on that list is ensuring that the emergency department's doctors aren't distracted by wayward teenagers. I think Dixie should have stepped in the first time Brackett bumped into Walters, and she should definitely have stepped in before he hung up with the squad (and yelled at her). It was definitely Dixie's job to ensure that the doctors have the tools and equipment they need to do their jobs efficiently and can focus fully on their patients. And if that means Dixie has to warn or even remove a meddling student, that's what she should have done. (In my opinion, anyway.)

On the call to the apartment's stuck elevator, I noticed that the engine rolled out of the station in front of the squad and we saw it go down the street that way, which was unusual. Also, I saw the same footage in this episode as in yesterday's ep, with the squad backing in and it looks like evening.

In that elevator scene, Kevin might have messed up a line or something, because he repeated a particular line twice. Once the hole is cut in the elevator roof, he says "we'll have to keep the EKG going while we move her up." Then the stokes is lowered into the 'vator and as they're putting her into it Roy says "we should keep the EKG going while we move her up." (Is there an echo in here??)

In the scene in the dorm, when Roy arrives and says "you're here early," if you look at the clock behind Johnny, it looks like it says 11:10 or so (hard to tell which hand is which). Then a minute later (but in the same scene), Johnny's again at the foot of the bed and the clock is behind him, it looks like it says 8:25. Now granted 8:25 makes more sense than 11:10, especially if each shift starts at 8:00, but it's funny that the time changed so radically so quickly.

Loved watching Johnny jump from rail car to rail car. It looks like a blast!

Also, I wonder what shoes Roy was shining at the station? (Note: the two tables were separated.) They don't really look like the type of work shoes they normally wear. Or are they? It's a little hard to tell as we don't usually get too good a look at them. Usually their shoes look like regular black shoes, but the ones Roy was shining were more workboot-looking, sturdy and with a small heel.

Oh, and about the nurse Walters drama... maybe in this first season, the PTB were still toying with the idea of having a heavy focus on the hospital, and if so they were going to need a larger group of characters (Early's interns, nursing students, etc.). Once they scrapped the soap opera idea, they just keep Morton (as a doctor) and eventually lose the baby-faced student nurse.

Lastly (I hope!) it's odd, in the final scene, that the entire shift of guys is hanging out at the station in their street clothes when they came on for their shift. In fact, it was *two* shifts of guys: the one going out (who should have been changing into street clothes) and "our" shift coming on--who should have been changing into their uniforms. What if a call came right then? The other shift would have to put in O.T.

* * *

Yes, I totally saw the student nurse's "flub" when she let go of the oxygen mask and it snapped onto old Sam's face. I think the scene had to be cut at that point because Nurse Walters started to laugh.

About the clothes they're wearing in that last scene.... I don't *think* the actors wore their own personal clothing, although it could be possible. I have to say I'm not always happy with the way Roy dresses. There are times when he looks like he should be plucking a guitar on Hee-Haw... they kind of make him wear these western-type clothes which I don't care for. I usually much prefer Johnny's look. But in this episode, in that final scene I thought Johnny didn't look so hot... I didn't like his shirt, and those off-white pants he was wearing were a little too tight and disco-ish for my tastes. Actually I didn't mind the shirt Roy was wearing (although the collar, while stylish at the time, was way too wide), but again, who dresses like that to go to work when all you're going to do once you get there is put on a uniform??? I think that Kirk guy looked the best.. But I just now noticed that there was a "wallet impression" on the back pocket of Roy's pants (jeans??), so maybe those *were* Kevin's own clothes?

Oh, and about Kevin's hair... I think his natural color was brown (-ish), as we see in later seasons when he no longer has to dye it. That darn Webb formula of "one dark-haired guy, one light-haired guy"!! Or to be fair, maybe it was just a Hollywood thing, and not just Webb (I shouldn't be so quick to blame him, I guess!). Anyway, once E! became a hit maybe the powers that be must have decided that it wouldn't kill the show if Kevin went back to his natural color. By then I think he had the right to insist on it.

~ ~ ~

I like this episode pretty well, all the rescues are interesting, if not outright thrilling.

The senior citizens in the elevator are interesting, watching Capt. Hammer and the paramedics figure out the best way to get the injured victims out of the 'vator. I was a bit surprised to see Chet handling the K-12; usually in the first season Stoker has been the go-to guy for the heavy equipment, since he's the one with 'real-world' experience. Also, we didn't see how they got the stokes out of the two-square-foot opening in the elevator, which could've been hairy, especially with the monitor and O2 tank included.

I noticed that they did have the old woman 'patched in,' you could see that her blouse was open below her bra area. (But of course, they didn't show the guys doing the actual patching-in.)

Continuity goof: Roy repeats twice the line about how she's "throwing PVCs, we should keep the EKG going while we get her out." I wonder which line was the scripted one?

I seem to remember mentioning this before but did anyone notice the crazy clock in the dorm during Johnny's bed-making scene? We see the clock once and it says one time, but in (supposedly) the same scene a few seconds later it's almost three hours earlier.

The junkman was funny, with his singed hair and face. And I had to chuckle when Roy told the guy to continue his story, saying, "Go on with your happening."

I've already expressed before my disdain for the Nurse Walters story; there is a review on the episode page of imdb which covers the ridiculousness of it. The scene of her standing like a goober while Brackett bumps into her not once, not twice, but *three* times... too ridiculous for words. And I blame Dixie.

I like the rescue at the railyard. It's so fun watching Johnny run along the tanker cars and jump from one to the next-- I bet that was a lot of fun to do, too. ;-) But the first victim, the one with limited exposure, got oxygen and an IV with D5W. The other victim, who'd been exposed a lot longer to stronger fumes, he didn't get any IV at all. In fact, he didn't even get a paramedic to accompany him to Rampart. *eyeroll* (And yet, Johnny and Roy were seen leaving the hospital and talking about the guy in the very next scene.)

This first season, in addition to seemingly always wearing their blue jackets (that trend continued in this ep), Johnny also doesn't say "Squad 51 available;" instead in this first season it's "Squad 51 returning to quarters." At least, most of the time.

*   *   *

I don't think Dixie would have told Nurse Walters anything too scandalous about Brackett... she knows how and when to keep secrets, I'm sure. She probably gave some sort of generic advice like "even though he's a doctor, he's just man, and he's not perfect either."   But as you say, we're probably supposed to wonder about that kind of 'girl talk' thing.

As for Cynthia getting Johnny's phone number... good point, I didn't even think of that.   I realize now that I didn't even mention this minor storyline in my earlier post, probably because I didn't think too much of it.   There were references to whether or not the girl was a 'dog,' (I think Roy said something that made it plain it was Johnny's word, as in 'is she what you would call a dog?') and also Johnny doesn't care for 'forward' women, hinting that a woman who calls men has to have something wrong with her.   Anyway, I just don't think I can muster up any annoyance at the chauvinistic attitude. We see it too often, unfortunately.

1.10 Hang-up

This episode was well-titled for a number of reasons, not the least of which is the fact that on at least three occasions there was some form of the phrase "hang up" spoken in dialogue (hang up, or hung up, etc.). And in both the physical and metaphorical sense.

First off, did we all notice the nameless, faceless new Captain? I don't think he was referred to by name, but imdb has the character listed as Capt. Hammer, so who knows? Meanwhile, the guys at Station 51 are watching Adam-12 (and didn't they look comfy in those horrible kitchen chairs?), and ironically in that particular A-12 episode, *both* Ron Pinkard and Marco

Lopez appear. (Speaking of Pinkard, I don't believe he was in this episode at all... at least, not as Dr. Morton.)

When Roy's talking to his wife on the phone to try to find out what happened in the episode, and then tells John what she said, I believe he says "Ann missed the rest of the show." Maybe he meant "and," or maybe he just skipped past the Jo part of JoAnn.

Anyway, in that scene at the station, while he's studying, both Roy and John are using green pens. For whatever that means....

When the lady with the headache is on the table for her spinal tap, she did look suitably worried and unhappy, and when she looked up to talk to Brackett, there's a real tear sliding down her face. Nice touch!

At the "industrial fire," the company name was Cosmo-Tec. It certainly was an industrial building, complete with a "hot-room" And yet... why were there people standing out in the streets in their robes and pajamas? Did they walk blocks from the nearest residential neighborhood, or is Cosmo-Tec messing with radiation materials in the middle of a suburban neighborhood?? (That street scene is going into the stock footage thread, too.) Speaking of that radiation thing, I wonder why the hospital can't or couldn't use one of their smaller out-buildings as a radiation 'hot zone' for cases like this? I realize that the situation probably doesn't arise very often (luckily!!!) but the building could be used for something else and double as a quarantine area, probably easier than scrubbing down the entire emergency department.

By the way, does anyone else get distracted by Dixie and her Amazing Lashes? The other day, between her and Nurse Walters, they probably had two feet of lashes going on. I wonder they could even blink from the weight of those things.

~ ~ ~

Okay, by my count (informal and non-binding) there were four mentions of some variation of the phrase "hung up." Just sayin'....

The ventilation burglar: the building he was in was a standard, boring office building. What was he stealing, paper clips and file folders? He said himself he 'travelled light' and didn't carry anything with him, so how did he get his loot (whatever it was) out of the building? Really, I don't think the writers put too much thought into this one. Whatever the "real" story in the logbook was, I have a feeling they left out some details to try to make it more interesting.

Did anyone see Johnny drop his helmet (accidentally) on Chet's head when he went up to look in the ductwork? Too funny!

At some point, didn't someone jokingly make a list of things the guys carry around with them? Whatever was on it, add a magic marker to the list. Both Roy and Captain What's-His-Name had markers they used to mark the ventilator.

According to the name badge, Deputy Vince's last name is Bronson; but I don't believe his last name is ever mentioned on the show (and his character is always listed as Vince or Officer Vince, with no last name).... The Ventilator Burglar has a severe case of Ketchup Blood; seriously, it was kinda pitiful-looking.... Did I imagine it or was Roy trying to get the burglar to quit talking in the ambulance? Every time he opened his mouth the guy incriminated himself further, and Roy told him to "take it easy."

I remember we talked before about this scene, but when Roy calls home to see if his wife watched the end of Adam-12, it sounds (and closed-captioning agrees) like he calls her Ann, instead of Joanne. And didn't someone mention a while back that during a mini-reunion of some E! actors, the name Joanne came up and Kevin asked "Who's Joanne?" LOLOL if true!!

The woman with the headache/aneurism: she always reminds me of Mackenzie Phillips from One Day at a Time. Also, I like the way she kind of gnawed on her finger while Brackett did the spinal tap; it looked pretty natural and real. And after Brackett told her he was sending her to a specialist, she says "Whatever." Sounded funny to me, because we tend to think of the "whatever" comment as a later phenomenon ('80s, valley girl, etc.).

I liked Dixie's little rant about her frustration with some of the people they have to deal with--it showed compassion for most, but impatience and anger with the 'takers' of the world. Brackett reminded her--and us--that emergency medicine was a new concept; nowadays we tend to forget that the specialty has only been around for 40-50 years.

The industrial fire: kind of ho-hum as far as I was concerned, with some weird continuity things. The company name was Cosmo-Tec Industries, which I find totally hilarious. Also, as I noted in a previous showing of this episode, I thought it was funny to see onlookers--wearing robes, no less--standing around an industrial fire. Doesn't every neighborhood have an industrial complex with radioactive materials?? (And since when does Dixie get Brackett's attention by calling "Dr. Brackett" rather than Kel? Guess they stuck by formal decorum in this early season.)

One thing I don't understand... the Battalion Chief said that "any equipment that goes in, stays in." Does that mean it's totally written off as contaminated, or can the equipment get decontaminated later on, like the FFs can? I wasn't clear on that.

Those six minutes they could spend in the hot room flew by awfully quick, didn't they? I swear, we saw the Cap and Chet in there, and it was literally only about 30 seconds.

Lastly, at the hospital, even with the radiation quarantine in effect, we still heard PA announcements for Treatment Room 6 or 2, or whatever. Weren't those treatment rooms the ones that were quarantined?? So where were they putting these patients?? Ah well, details, details....

* * *

> The Book says the rescue of the burglar in the air duct was filmed in a sound stage so I guess that's why that office seemed so boring.

Actually, I was wondering what there was to steal in *any* office building? Unless there was a jewelry store on the ground floor, I don't think there would be much of interest for anyone to take. :) Plus, as I said, how would he escape with loot, if he traveled so light via the air ducts? He said he didn't carry anything on him ("not even a toothpick") because he didn't have room.

> Did anyone else want to just smack the guy with the broken leg? Ugh!
> And every episode this season we hear that "stat ident doctor" page. Did we ever determine what or who that is?

YES, I wanted to smack that surfer dude into next week. >:(

As for "Stat Ident Doctor," I don't think we ever came up with a definitive answer. Someone posited that it was a way of saying "will the doctor in Room 3 (or whatever) identify himself." Maybe to keep up with which doctor sees which patient?? I dunno. It's another E! mystery. ;-)

1.11 Crash

First off, it occurred to me that this episode might have the scene that Randy talked about in his interview, with them being "up in the trees" working on someone who'd been in a plane crash, and Kevin wrapping someone's head in gauze. But I'm doubting that story, for a couple of reasons which I'll get to shortly.

First off, Johnny's ticked off at Roy and Roy doesn't know why. After they brought the burglar-slash-heart-patient into the hospital and Gage gets snippy in the treatment room, Dr. Early says "What's with him?" and Roy basically replies "h3ll if I know," and he picks up the O2 and leaves the room to go back to the squad. In the following scene (after a commercial break) we see Roy come out of the hospital to the squad but.... the oxygen tank is gone. All he's carrying is the handy-talkie. I hope they don't need the oxygen again anytime soon.

The babysitter who brings in the overdosed boy is played by Bobby Troupe's daughter. She's the same one who's in at least one other episode, with the "host of golden daffodils."

Now, onto the tree-top plane rescue.... It's obvious that there was real footage used, out there on the hill, with people up in the trees, etc. I did wonder how both John and Roy are able to climb the rope into the tree...*without* gloves. Wouldn't that hurt like crazy??

Also, obviously the scenes of John and Roy working on the plane were filmed on a set. When Johnny calls out from his perch on the branch, you can hear echoes; it sounds very much like a soundstage. And, as Roy is joining Johnny on the conveniently large branch, you can see three wires off to the right-hand side.

In that airplane scene, there's a character who Roy bandaged around his head, but in his interview I thought Randy mentioned that the victim was a woman whose head Roy was bandaging, but in this episode it was a man, and we really didn't see more than just a bit of it. Also, if this scene was indeed filmed on a set, Kevin wouldn't have had any reason to be afraid of the height. Kevin himself has said that heights didn't bother him until season three or so, so I doubt a first-season episode would show it.

By the way, the house with the burglar/heart-patient in it... that house also appeared in an episode of Adam-12. Another bizarre coincidence-- last week I saw William Katt in an episode of E!, and on that very same day, Barbara Hale and her hubby (can't recall the name) were on Adam-12 episode that aired that same day. Those two are William Katt's parents, so the entire family was on TV on the same day, albeit on different shows.

* * *

About Roy (Kevin) mouthing the words over the HT, it made me think of something. Bear with me a minute on this, as I veer off into another topic for a moment.

On Adam-12, we (the audience) hear the dispatcher's voice over the car radio, and Reed will pick up the radio and reply "One Adam-12, roger." But while they were filming those car scenes, there was no voice over the radio. Instead, a script supervisor* would be lying on the floor of the backseat reading all the dispatcher's lines. (The actual dispatcher's voice would later be dubbed in.) In this way, the actors could time their response to when the script person spoke, as if speaking directly to the dispatcher.

How does that tie in with Roy mouthing the dispatcher's words at Rampart? Well, what if there really was no voice (Sam Lanier's or anyone else's) coming over the HT when they supposedly get calls? Just like on Adam-12, the dispatcher's voice could be dubbed in later, but the difference is, in this scene on E!, there's no place for anyone to hide to read the dispatcher's lines, so Kevin would have to time his response very carefully. Maybe he was mouthing the words as a way to judge how long it would take "Sam" to read off his call, so he'd know when to "respond." It probably is *not* the case, and while it is within the realm of possibility, it still doesn't explain Kevin mouthing John's words in the locker room in the other episode. So maybe it's just something Kevin did now and then.

But it makes you wonder also if that's how they deal with filming the calls at the station. There could have been someone offstage who rang a bell or hit a buzzer to "stand in" for the tones and the call, and the actors reacted to nothing. Then the call would be plugged in later. It would explain the times when Mike runs to the map before we hear the address, or when all the guys run out of the kitchen/rec room when it's a call for "only" the squad, etc.

* Interesting trivia: the script supervisor for Adam-12 (there were more than one, but the one who was there the longest) was Cynnie Troup, Bobby Troup's other daughter. She really did lie on the floor of the Adam-12 car as it was being towed around LA, and she really did speak the lines of the dispatcher. (Wouldn't that be the coolest job *ever???*) After Adam-12 ended, she went on to work on a lot of other TV shows.

~ ~ ~

Last episode of Season One. For the record, I believe this ep is the last we'll see Nurse Ellen Bart; I wonder why they didn't continue with her. Eventually she and John might have made a good couple... once he matured a little. (Also, I think we'll only see student nurse Sharon Walters one or two more times. Her, I won't really miss; she's cute but I can do without her.) Speaking of nurses, at some point didn't someone mention nurses' capes? I don't think we ever saw any in season one. Were there any in the pilot? Or were the capes pretty much passé by then?

~ Episode opens with the ambulance arriving at Rampart and Johnny bringing in a young football player. Incidentally, this is the scene in which Johnny put his hand up to protect himself from Decapitation Corner. I could have sworn it was Roy who did it... maybe he does at some point, and I haven't seen it yet.

~ Cecily Tyson is the boy's annoying mother. Her character's name is Joanne, oddly enough.

~ On the drive to the heart-attack burglar, we see the 'old' squad driving down the road, but when the guys turn in to the driveway, it's the 'correct' model. By the way, the wife-burglar apparently went outside and flagged down a passing plumber when her husband fell ill. What, that nice house they were ripping off didn't have a phone?? Why didn't *she* just call the fire department? Better yet, why not just call an ambulance, maybe then the cops might not have showed up. (I'm still not sure why they showed up anyway.)

~ The scene when Roy confronts Johnny outside the Emergency entrance: toward the end of their talk, you see a hospital worker (Angelo DeMeo) exit from the building and pass Roy and Johnny. After they leave, the action moves inside the hospital where, in the *same scene* when Nurse Walters is talking to Dr. Early in the hallway--who should be seen pushing a wheelchair but orderly Angie DeMeo. He leaves the hospital one minute and is back to work the next. Or maybe he mastered the art of bilocation.

~ When Dixie was talking to her step-daughter--er, I mean, the babysitter who brought in the boy, you can hear a page in the background: "Dr. Brackett, Dr. Brackett." And that's it. There is no more to the page, all it did was call to Brackett.

~ When my cat is being particularly crazy, I tell her, "You're a nut. But you're a friendly kind of nut."

~ We briefly see Chet in this ep, in the day-room/break-room of the station, but nobody else from Engine 51. There is the scene with Captain Smith/VanOrden/Whatever giving the KMG-365 for them--once--but generic scenes like that are almost always stock footage; it could have been filmed at any time. (Although he is credited for this Crash episode.)

~ I had to laugh because Firefighter Kirk is now Paramedic Kirk again. And he no longer works at 51s, but at 110s, with Wheeler. Maybe he's been cloned: the FF works at 51 and the PM works at 110s.

~ Funny how the guys tend to refer to other fire stations and add an "s" to the end. 51s... 110s... 99s, etc.

~ In general I'm not fond of the plane-in-a-tree rescue, for one because it's very obvious that the tree-top scenes are filmed in the studio, and that pulls me out of the moment every time. I did notice that while still on the ground, all the guys wore gloves when working with the ropes, but did not wear them when they climbed. It's been a long time since I handled anything rougher than a clothesline, but I think I remember it hurting. Firefighters' hands must be one huge callous.

So... bring on Season Two!

Season Two

Big changes this season:

~ Hello, Captain Stanley! No fanfare, not even an introduction, he's just there on our screen in the very first scene. And we're all glad.

~ Chet's hair, on both his head and his face. He's ditched the LACoFD-approved short, side-parted hair and is letting his hair grow. And there's also the 'stache.

~ I know we've only seen one ep of this season so far, but so far I've seen scant presence of the blue jackets. Personally I find that good news. :)

~ Another change is at Rampart: the big, bulky tape machine in the base station is gone, replaced by a smaller and sleeker version. No more big tapes for Nurse Walters to unspool.

~ Still at Rampart, the elevator is here! At the end of the hallway by the base station, what was just a generic door last season is now an elevator. My psychic abilities tell me it will remain an elevator for seasons to come. *wink*

~ Oh, one more change with 'the guys'.... Johnny's funky leather watch-strap is history. He and Roy both have new watches. I assume they were LACoFD issue, or at least approved. Otherwise, why would they be identical?

2.1 Decision/Problem

Yaaaayyyy!!! This was one of the major "Big Issues" episodes that we all love, probably the "biggest" one of the series. It's also the first ep of the 2nd season. Here are some thoughts in general:

~ In the engine-crushing rescue, couldn't you have just smacked that neighbor lady?? Johnny should have put her in her place and told her to "shut up" so he could hear on the biophone.

~ First episode with Cap Stanley... wonder why they didn't make a mention about the "new" captain who transferred in from some other station. And also the first appearance of Chet's mustache.

~ At the first rescue, when they got the engine off the guy, Marco and Mike were holding the engine up with the chain. Then they came to help the others, but we don't know what they did with the chains. Tie them off? Hand them off to some guys on the set? I wonder why they didn't just lower the engine to the floor.

~ That stupid antenna thing on the ambulance (the one that fell off), of course we've never seen it before, because it's never been important before. Seemed like kind of a flimsy arrangement for a vehicle that literally deals with life and death situations.

~ I know Johnny stayed back to deal with the upset wife (if he hadn't, he would have seen the antenna fall off), but when he did drive the squad to the hospital, why didn't he come across the ambulance? I guess they weren't stopped long enough.

~ That thing that Brackett told Roy, about "you need to ask yourself am I the most qualified person available to help".... I believe Roy repeats that line in a future episode. Maybe with one of the paramedic trainees they have to deal with?? Can't recall when, but I know he does.

~ That house fire, the final call... did everyone notice the neighbors in their robes and pajamas? That same scene/footage was used the other day in the industrial fire, the building with the radioactive material. Funny that this instance of it aired so close to the first one, which was a different season. And I believe we'll probably see it again in the future.

~ Seems to me this episode showed more of the "stuff" that the firefighters do: men manning hoses, an engineer (not Stoker) adjusting the dials and hoses, etc. Maybe in the 2nd season the show got a boost in their budget and they decided to showcase their operations and how they do their jobs a little bit.

~ I practically laughed out loud when Roy was in the house looking for the little boy. Did anyone notice the flashlight he was using, and how there was no light coming from it? He was flashing it around and there was *no* light.. (Reminded me of the police station on Adam-12... no glass in the doors or the 'windows.'

And lastly... who can forget the beautiful sight of two tired, dirty, sooty firefighters in the squad driving back to the station. I know it's strange, but I find that so... appealing. Sure, guys, I'll help you clean up; let me sponge you off....

* * *

Oh, I just remembered... did anyone notice the funny time-warp thing with the bull? I think they tried to make it look like the bull was moving faster than it was, and they sped up the film. It looked pretty cheesy.

~ ~ ~

Not sure why there's confusion or alternate titles for this episode. They both represent the gist of the storyline.

Anyway, I do like this one, because it's one of the first (and strongest, and best) of the Issues episodes. Some heartfelt soul-searching going on in LA County in this one.

On the way to the first call, they passed some Quonset huts. I don't recall seeing them for quite a while up until now. (Also, I noticed that when Roy had the ambulance resume their trip to the hospital, they were right in front of the granary.)

We have a strong contender in the Stupid Neighbor contest. I really wanted to slap that woman. She must've said "this is terrible" about fifteen times.

Did anyone else hear some sort of racket or noise as both the squad and engine pulled up to the scene on that fallen-engine call? Sort of sounded like they brushed up against some trash cans or ran over something (like plastic bottles, although I'm sure that wasn't the case).

So the guy got pinned down by the fallen engine. One question: where were his legs and feet? When they're moving the car, someone says "watch his legs," but I can only assume his legs are either tucked into the engine compartment, or poking out the bottom beneath the car, and thus had to be 'watched' while they moved the car.

I think this was mentioned before, but after they hoisted the engine off the guy, Stoker and Lopez were holding it up with the chains. Then all of a sudden the end of the chains is off-screen and we see Mike and Marco do something else. Guess they handed the chain over to the prop guys, maybe?

What can we say about Dr. Sunderland? I half expected him to have a waxed mustache to twirl. Even though I've seen this ep a number of times before, the irony of something just hit me in this viewing. When he and Brackett were butting heads about treatment, Sunderland called the man "my patient." Brackett replied that "until he gets through those doors, he's *my* patient." So as it happened, when he was Brackett's patient (and the paramedics' patient) he was brought into the hospital alive; once he was there, it was while he was under *Sunderland's* care that the man died. (Is it wrong that I felt a little bit of satisfaction at that fact??)

After Sunderland dressed him down, did anyone notice Roy sort of turning away, his back to the camera? That must be something he unconsciously does when he's upset. He does almost the exact same thing in Trainee after he reams out Ed Marlowe in the locker room at the station.

Funny, when Roy and Johnny got back to the station and Johnny checked the map to see where Roy stopped, and how far he was from the hospital, etc., he wasn't pointing anywhere near where he looked before they went on the run, when he checked the map for the address.

Like last time, I have to laugh when I see the scene with the bull. For one thing, I don't think we see both the squad and the bull in the same shot at any time. And for another thing, the footage of the bull was obviously sped up to make it look like he was moving faster than he was. It was too funny. Only in '70s TV shows, right? The producers probably said "Eh, nobody will see it clearly, or remember it very well."
^ ^
–

Again in this episode, we hear pages for people, with no instructions. One was just as everyone was leaving the Treatment Room after the doctor died ("Dr. Early, Dr. Early"). Another one was for "Miss McCall, Miss McCall." Oddly, I think it was during her "I'm tired and whipped" speech, or at the end of it. But it's odd to hear the pages like that. Maybe Rampart's PA system is haunted, paging phantom doctors to Emergency that we never see (Jose

Estrada), and now calling out to the doctors we know for no apparent reason.

2.2 Kids

This episode should be titled "Kids (or, in Johnny's words, "I'm glad I'm not married!")

Mrs. Gentry, the abused kid's mom, appears in a number of E! episodes. We saw her in Botulism, as the wife of the first botulism victim, the guy at the movie studio. This episode touched on another sad trend of the times (early '70s): that women wouldn't leave their (abusive) husbands, not because they love the jerk, but because they needed someone to 'take care of' them. A lot of women with kids didn't work in those days, so leaving their husbands meant they'd have no money, and the women probably didn't have much in the way of work skills or experience either. (Yes, I realize I'm generalizing... my own mother worked at least part-time since the early '60s, but most of my friends' mothers stayed home.)

Boy, get a load of Brackett's groovy suit, with the wide lapels, extra-wide tie, and whatever that Velcro-looking stuff was on the pockets.

Cute, watching Boot with Roy. Kevin did seem very comfortable with the dog. And in the hiker rescue scene, John had to move Boot before he could rappel down the cliff, as Boot's paws were straddling his line. It was cute! (And if I didn't already know, I wouldn't have recognized John Travolta. He just looked like a dark-haired kid, like a thousand others. The voice is pretty recognizable, though.)

Oh, about Boot... I saw an episode of The Virginian a while back which actually starred Boot. Boot was the dog's real name and he had a big role in that show.

Here we are in the 2nd season, and along with the obvious changes (new captain, Chet's mustache), there's another change... Johnny's groovy brown leather watch is gone, and he now wears a "big-boy" watch. Also, when they leave Rampart they're still calling in with "Squad 51, in quarters." I think they must quit that pretty soon though.

Hmmm, no Marco or Mike in this one. You'll notice in the scene where they're called out to the brush fire, we see "people" running to the engine, but it's nobody we recognize. Obviously footage of the 'real' firefighters from 127s.

~ ~ ~

Good news: Boot comes to visit!! Bad news: He doesn't stay. Boo.

~ At the scene of the boy stuck in the hole, his little friend was wearing a red and white gingham-checked shirt. So the trend starts early, apparently....

~ Also at that scene, Johnny/Randy really did get all dirty. You can see him shake the dirt out of his hair once the others have the little boy safe. (And good continuity for a change, as his shirt doesn't magically appear clean immediately afterward; instead, it stays dirty for a couple of scenes.)

~ The kid with head stuck in basement frame: once again, this is a scene that's a little similar to a scene in Adam-12. In that show, though, a kid had his head stuck between pickets of an iron fence. But anyway, this one was cute, and the guys were good with the little kid, especially Johnny. Btw, that house kind of reminded me of the house where the guys treated a dog-bite and Johnny found out that his g.f. Valerie had kids. (Also: when Johnny first squats down to check on the boy, you can clearly see the mic-pack taped to his back.)

~ Speaking of what's in Johnny's shirt (mmmm!), it's true that the "object" is already making regular appearances in his front pocket. Bad Randy, for not staying in character!!

~ This was another Issues episode, but it was Brackett's issue. It also served as a PSA. During the hearing or whatever legal thing that was in the Family Court, why didn't the woman (I assume she was some sort of county attorney) why didn't *she* ask Frankie any questions? Yes, he would probably have lied to help his mother, but it might have been obvious that he was lying, and that might have swayed the judge in some way.

~ I have to note that the judge flubbed it after he gave his ruling in favor of the parents. He said "Court is recessed," when what he should have said is "Court is adjourned." A recess is a temporary break in proceedings, but when a case is 'closed,' court is adjourned. (I've been watching a lot of Perry Mason.)

~ We see more 'real' FFs today, both responding at the station to their respective vehicles, and also when leaving the station, when the cameraman is on top of the Crown.

~ At the final rescue, with the lost hikers, the one hiker is walking *toward* the squad, and then says he lost sight of his friend a while back. So what does Johnny do? He walks up the road in the direction the squad just came... the opposite direction from where the guy had been. There's no way Vinnie Barbarino could have been where Gage was looking for him. Good thing Boot has a good nose, right?

~ ~ ~

One thing that this episode brings to mind for me isn't really specific to Emergency, but more an observation of the times. Up until the mid-'70s or so, many women viewed marriage as a safety net, a means of providing herself with comfort and financial security. How often in movies/shows of the '50s and '60s do we hear mention of a woman who has "marriage on her mind," or that "she's looking for a husband"? Entire movies were written back in the day about women on the hunt for men to marry. They wanted to secure themselves a home and family, someone to 'take care of them'... and love wasn't necessarily a requirement. In this episode of E!, Mrs. Gentry never said she stayed with her %$@! of a husband because she loved him, instead she said "we have nowhere to go, nobody to take care of us." (Or words to that effect.) In other words, she probably only married the jerk in the first place because he could provide a home for herself and her son.

The same concept can be seen from time to time in Adam-12 as well, which of course began in the late '60s, and overlapped with Emergency! for a few years. In one instance Malloy and Reed answer a call from a woman who claims her husband hit her (they were mainly just arguing and she called the cops out of spite). But when Reed discovered there was a previous warrant out for the man, the cops have to take him into custody. Wifey says, "that old warrant is from me, but I want to drop the charges, don't arrest him." Malloy replies, "Too late, we have to take him." And she says, "You're going to leave me here? What am I going to do? I'm only a woman." (Grrr. Sorry, it sets my teeth on edge to even type that last comment.)

Then, another time Reed suggests (for the millionth time) that Malloy should get married. His reasons: Pete wouldn't have to go home to an empty apartment... he could have hot meal ready for him when he walks in the door... he'd have companionship. Do you believe that?? Those are the reasons for men to marry. What a deal!! Men get someone to cook and clean for them, and women get someone to cook *for*. Yeah, *that's* why we get married, isn't it??? Might as well be the 1860s rather than the 1960s.

Anyway, these days, I don't think we hear too many women (young or er, more mature) who say they want to marry just to get a roof over their heads. Women today are more likely to pick up a hammer and nails and build their own roof rather than marry the first guy they meet who has a decent job. The more I watch these old shows the more I realize how limiting life was (for many people, not all) back in the day. And the thing is, it was so ingrained in people that these ideas were accepted unquestioningly. Marry young, marry for comfort and security, make the best of it no matter what.

Whew! Sorry for the rant, I just had to get that off my chest. I feel better now. At least, until I run across another example of this antiquated thinking.

2.3 Show Biz

Show Biz... I noticed Johnny's wearing his holster on his left side in this one. Someone mentioned that earlier (first season) and it's still true, although somewhere along the way he does switch it to right side.

When treating Dr. Knott ("with a K"), Johnny puts the O2 on his face and then replaces the doctor's hat on his head. It's so cute how he does that, he tilts the hat to keep the sun out of the doctor's eyes. Just like yesterday he had to move Boot's butt off his rope.

For the drowning call... maybe it's just me, but I'd think the paramedics (or at least *one* of them) would have run ahead to check out the situation first before taking the time to get all the gear out of the squad. Drowning is like a fire--you wait too long and there's nobody to rescue. Anyway, when dealing with this guy, I noticed his "southern belle" wife had a very unusual-looking ring on, sort of like a large orange ball. (Orange, in case that colored font is hard to read.) Anyway, it was pretty odd and unique, I thought.

The ring might be odd, but apparently it was popular, because one of the models at the photo shoot was wearing the *exact same ring*. Right down to the orange color. Maybe there was a sale on them at Woolworth's, so the wardrobe people bought a bunch of them.

At Rampart, Dr. Knott is in his bed (no roommate, luckily)... he makes a dumb move and the catheter breaks off (should they really be that easy to break??). Anyway, Nurse Carol runs out of the room for help and... she's in the Emergency Department! Apparently the door is a magic portal, because on one side it's a semi-private hospital room, and on the other side is the Rampart hallway we see with all the treatment rooms. It's magic!!

There were a couple of calls for "Stat Ident doctor" and "Dr. Jose Estrada" today. I think I noticed at least one of each.

The stunt guy rescue with the wagon... he said his legs were numb and he couldn't feel anything below his waist, but in the shot of the wagon falling off the cliff, you can see his legs moving. Also, when they're getting ready to strap him into the stokes, the drug box is right next to him (dangerously close, I thought). Sure enough, as the chopper begins to lift the stokes, it knocks the drug box over. I sure hope it's waterproof.

Another bold Brackett fashion statement in the last scene: wide-striped pants and a wide patterned tie. Yikes! And it seemed to me like one second Brackett and Early were talking about something, and the next second Dixie (at the base station) knew what they were talking about. Maybe Rampart also enhances mental telepathy in addition to hosting magic portals.

Lastly, the conversation with John and Roy was funny after that rescue, when they were talking about how "Hollywood is strange," or whatever the exact words were. Roy says "We take as many chances as they do," and John says "Yeah, but we're paid for it." Layer upon layer upon layer of meaning for this show.

~ ~ ~

Or, The One Where Johnny Meets Beautiful Models. Although later on he didn't seem all that impressed for some reason, and complained that they were 'too skinny.' This, from the same guy who seems to reject the idea of going out with any woman who weighs more than 150. Wait 'til you're 40 years old, John Gage, and you'll call those 150-lb women skinny, too. In any case, I like this episode, I think it has a little of everything. Only complaint (minor one) is that we don't see much of the rest of the guys away from the station.

The show opens with R and J and Chet in the locker room/bathroom cleaning, but when the tones sound, we see them magically leaving the dayroom. Station 51 features teleportation--who knew!!

~ We see the trestle bridge in this one! Is this the trestle's debut, or have we seen it in any earlier episodes?

~ Ya gotta love Dr. Knott, with a K. He's cute and, unlike so many other one-time characters on this show, he's not extremely annoying. This show's writers had such a habit of inserting stereotypes and extremes into the show that it was nice to have a character you didn't want to strangle or roll your eyes about.

~ It was cute when Johnny took off Dr. Knott's hat to put the O2 on him, and then he replaced the Doc's hat, to keep the sun out of his eyes. :)

~ Why did the lady (wife of the guy who almost drowned in the pool) have a southern accent? Do that many southerners relocate to Los Angeles that we run into them on a regular basis? And what was with her outfit? Personally I thought she was a little old to wear that... although she *was* in her own back-yard, so I guess she's allowed. By the way, why was Johnny explaining the medical stuff to her at Rampart? It looked kind of weird and it's not his job.

~ Did anyone note the large orange round-ball ring she was wearing?

~ Why would the writers have Roy reference Chester Morris? Even back in the day I don't think I ever heard of him. I had to look him up. (P.S.: he was an actor.)

~ Dr. Knott with a K looked like he was in a patient room, but when the nurse stepped out it looked like she was in the Emergency Department hallway.

~ During the photo shoot, that was Hal Frizzell (stunt guy and all-around orderly/ambulance driver) who played the photographer. And the one model who put make-up on Johnny was wearing that same ugly orange round-ball ring that the other woman wore. (And the other model was wearing Miss Jane Hathaway glasses.)

~ For the final call, must be weird to drive through a movie lot that looks like a real city, but there's no traffic. Also, at the site of the overturned coach, I was a little surprised they didn't tie off the coach to the engine rather than having two or three guys holding it. (eye-roll icon)

~ I'm assuming the crane came back and got either Roy or Johnny to go in the ambulance, since they did start an IV on the guy. We see the squad and engine return to the station at the same time, which would be unlikely if the squad went to Rampart. But this show does have magic, so.... who knows.

2.4 Virus

This is one of those episodes which, if you ask 100 fans—female fans, to be precise—their top 3 episodes, this would probably be one of them. Most likely Snakebite and The Nuisance would be the other two. Why, you ask?? Because they form the JIJT... the "Johnny in Jeopardy" Triumvirate. This show's fans, especially women, love it when John Gage is hurt or in danger.

Anyway, more about the theme of the show in a bit. First, a few small trivia details....

~ The man who played Jenny's father (the virus girl), that actor also played the used-car salesman who was trapped in the car with the tiger.

~ I noticed a little more Webb-speak in this episode (sadly). Mainly on the building roof-top as they were discussing how to get their cardiac victim off the scaffolding. (P.S., you can see the 'victim' holding onto the underside of the scaffolding with his left hand after Johnny attached his carabiner and is about to pass out.)

~ At the station, when John and Roy are talking next to the squad about Jenny, it clearly looks as if the engine is gone, there's a lot of room next to where they're standing in the apparatus room. Then the call comes in for the boy stuck in tree, and as the squad leaves the station, we see the engine there as well. It just appeared out of nowhere!

~ For the man on scaffold call, Station 51 was called as well as Truck 210. On the roof, some of the 210 guys were helping with the ropes, and their helmets were different from 51's helmets. The guy's number on the helmet was red on black. (And I was relieved to see they were wearing gloves as they worked the ropes.)

~ At the hospital, Roy goes to tell Morton that Dr. Early needs him (Morton had just told the fireman's wife that he'd died). When Morton is leaving that scene, he hesitates, as if unsure whether he should exit via the "elevator" or through the door Roy had come through. He took the door. But it looked as if Ron Pinkard didn't know which he was supposed to do.

~ Dixie made a reference to Roy about his "partner" waiting for him in the squad, and Roy qualified that as "my *temporary* partner." So we know he was working with someone. But at the end, when he went to see Johnny in the last scene, we clearly see Roy backing the squad in at the emergency entrance, and he's alone in the vehicle. Clearly a stock shot, from a scene in which Johnny had ridden to Rampart in the ambulance, but still, it's a boo-boo because there would never be a lone paramedic on duty.

Now, on to my main problem with this episode... Knowing what the doctors knew, or at the very least, strongly suspected, that Jenny had a communicable virus, that it might have involved the monkey, that a number of people, including Roy and John, had come into contact with them... the doctors did NOT take Roy and John off duty. Instead, knowing *full well* they'd been exposed, the two paramedics were allowed to work, when at any time they could be taken ill, or, even worse, treat patients in very close proximity, thus putting *them* in danger as well. Shame on the doctors! Also, shame on Gage, for knowing he felt so tired, and on the roof even felt a little hinky, and yet he didn't take himself out of the game. He knew he'd been exposed, and he knew he didn't feel 100%, he should have added 2+2 and even if he didn't get 4, he should have erred on the side of caution. It's possible (maybe not likely or provable, but *possible*) that if Johnny had stepped aside and let Roy go down to the scaffold to begin with, Roy might have gotten to the man in time and been able to save him. Instead the man died. Those extra five minutes could have saved him. It would have been better, in the long run (and much more realistic) if later on Johnny had expressed remorse and/or grief about that situation. But I realize this show wants and needs to have a nice uplifting ending, so that didn't happen. However, in real life, it would have almost certainly have affected Johnny, and it would have been another good "issue" for this show to deal with.

~ ~ ~

This is the first of the JIJ trifecta. However, I'm going to skip a lot of the virus-related stuff because I find it a little unbelievable.

~ I like the boy-in-the-tree rescue, even though the scenes inside the treehouse were obviously a set. But it was good. Except for when Johnny supposedly threw up the line (rope) to Roy--no way he could have thrown that rope that far (I don't think), and Roy/Kevin obviously just picked up a rope that had been set nearby.

~ When the engine got there, Cap called out, "DeSoto, you got a line up there?" and Roy answered "Yo." I thought that was so cute and funny for some reason.

~ Would the hospital really allow a student nurse to work with a virulent communicable disease that was as yet unidentified, much less untreatable?? I strongly doubt it. (Are student nurses allowed in the hospital sites in Texas dealing with Ebola? Doubt it.)

~ Knowing how important it was, and how high the stakes were, I find it inconceivable (and practically criminal) that Jenny didn't think of mentioning "Roger" sooner. Duh!

~ I think it's been discussed before, but was it mentioned on the show *how* Brackett got infected? Not only did he take 'precautions' while handling Koki, but he fell ill *before* Johnny did.

~ Speaking of time, the virus must have had a 2-day incubation period, because in the scene at the station Roy says that "the lab" has been working on identifying the virus for "48 hours straight." Which makes me wonder--again--why Brackett fell ill before Johnny did.

~ Speaking of Johnny falling ill, I'm going to skip the part where he's even on duty and treating patients, and that he himself had a dizzy spell but didn't say anything. (eye-roll) But when he's on that scaffolding it must have been quite a leap of faith (or *fall* of faith, as the case may be) for Randy to allow himself to roll off that scaffolding. And while it's possible that was a stunt double, it did kind of look like Randy.

2.5 Peace Pipe

I agree with those who feel that Johnny is right to feel offended at Chet's comments. I did have the feeling that Chet was purposely goading Johnny right from the beginning (or as Roy noted, 'baiting' him), but that doesn't make it better (or right). And yeah, I was a little surprised at Roy's comment... although sometimes Johnny *is* a little too sensitive. (reference the "you're a nut" conversation).

I'm a little curious about the whole Indian theme of this episode. I wonder where that came from? Having it come up once or twice at the station would have been one thing, but for it to run throughout the whole episode seemed a little much. Johnny's diatribe about the anthropologists seemed to take the topic to a whole different level, as if the writers were trying to make a definite point. But I don't know why... solely for Randy's benefit? Far as I know, he didn't grow up on a reservation and may never have experienced anything along those lines (although I could be wrong about that). So I'm not sure why they thought it was important enough to make a mini "after school special" about it.

At the scene of the drunk-driver accident, I totally agree with you about the mother constantly yelling her child's name. "Debbie! Debbie!" (And yes, Harold Perrineau's character on Lost came to my mind too!! Not only did he yell "Waaaalt" numerous times, but if I had a nickel for every time he referred to Walt as "my boy," I could take us all out to dinner.) Anyway, it seems to me that I heard somewhere (maybe an interview?) that in these scenes, a lot of dialogue wasn't written out, so victim/actors kind of took whatever guidelines they had and did what they could with it. So lacking other direction (or 'motivation,' as the old show-biz trope goes) the actor just repeats the dialogue they do have and milk it for all it's worth. I noticed something similar with the annoying neighbor lady in Problem.

Another rescue has the paramedics on a scaffold that's under fire from a sniper. They didn't know until they got up there that the victim had been shot, and of course they didn't get shot at themselves until they were up on the scaffolding, either. So at that point there was no point in going back down without their victim. (Although why Cap said "Squad 51 available," I don't know. Especially since they left the drug box on the scaffolding when they came down.)

I didn't notice that particular sound error you mention (even though I listen with headphones), but I did notice a different one in that same "house-fire" call. Inside the house, after Johnny runs out of the house and Roy is inside, Roy looks disgustedly at the hose and says "what's coming out of this hose?" It's Roy standing there, and Roy's mouth is moving, but it's definitely not Roy's voice we hear. It's Johnny's.

I too recognized Kip Niven, the little girl's dad. One of his other appearances on E! is as a paramedic trainee. I think he's the one who's good, but doesn't have a lot of confidence. (I believe he coughed a lot after exposure to smoke??)

Also, for the final rescue on the building, when we see the engine and squad driving there (and other scenes of the street), you can tell the street was blocked off for filming. There are too many people just standing on sidewalk along the street--if it had been 'real,' everyone would be walking one place or another. But everyone was standing around, just wanting to see the filming. At least, that was my impression.

~ ~ ~

This topic could be added to the list of Things to Ask in Interviews Someday. I wonder why this episode was written and what Randy thought of the title topic of this episode.

~ The first accident, with "Debbie! Debbie! Debbie!" Seriously, do people think that constantly calling their loved one's name is going to help? (I shouldn't talk; thank heaven I've never been in a situation like that, but I like to think logic would be instinctive and I wouldn't be so annoying and distracting to those who are trying to help.) Anyway, I guess the FD really does just hose down gasoline spills (we discussed this in the ep about the gas-station spill).

~ No sooner do the cops and the fire department arrive on scene of this accident, than the tow truck got there right behind them. Wha— ?? That never happens.

~ In a previous episode (1st season) Vince the deputy's last name was Bronson. In this one it's Smith.

~ At the station that scene was funny when Johnny was talking to Chet and gesturing with the huge knife. Roy finally took it away from him. That book Chet had was titled The Problemed Indian, by Marcus Parkham. (Not a real book or author, that I can find.)

~ I know the girdle scene is usually a fan favorite, but I find it a little ridiculous. If a girdle can be fastened, it can be *un*fastened. I assume that would have been tried first. (Fun fact: the building that rescue was in, I think we see it again-- see them drive up to it--in another episode coming up.)

~ The fuel in the toilet: kind of funny, certainly not as bad as it could have been. I still don't think it sounds like Roy who says "What the heck is coming out of this hose," but I'll let that lie. One thing I definitely noticed was the background noise with the sound of a tape being rewound or something, sort of that "zzzzzt" sound that tape recorders used to make. For those of you playing at home, it occurs right after the man sets the lawn on fire with his cigarette, just as Johnny's putting his turnout on.

~ At the scene on the roof, Cap calls in a Code L, which is for law enforcement. Kind of redundant since he already told dispatch to contact the sheriff about the gunman.

~ Speaking of the shooter: he was behind Roy and Johnny, but Cap tells the other guys of 51 to take cover too, even though they're not in any immediate danger where they are.

~ And again we all noticed they left the drug box up on the scaffold. But I find it odd that Roy talks about how much blood the guy has lost and they have to get him down asap, but once they get the vic down to the roof they didn't even treat him, much less give him an IV (which is when they'd have noticed the drug box). In fact, Cap called in that both the engine and squad were available... instead of them going to Rampart with the victim.

2.6 Saddled

I agree with the assessment of the bus-crash victim: I bet the "real" call from the log didn't involve a beautiful 26-year-old nun... only in Hollywood!! And your use of "beatific" was appropriate too. There was even a tear! I do like that prayer, the Memorare. I didn't learn it in Catholic school* but I'm familiar with it now.

I too liked Roy being the focus of this one. But I have to laugh... this isn't the first show I've seen in which a character protests "I'm not Catholic." You don't have to be Catholic in order to read a prayer, or listen to someone recite one. Yes, the rescue was a little heavy-handed with the religious stuff, but since this show never usually 'went there,' and it was a one-time thing, it's forgivable. (Although I was confused... I assumed one of the paramedics, most likely Roy, would have gone to Rampart with her anyway; they established an IV so they had to do the follow-up to the hospital. Right?? But then, I guess she couldn't have asked Roy to go with her so she wouldn't be afraid. *hack* Pardon me, just OD'ing on a little on all the saccharine.)

Ronne Troup was the girl with the injured eye. Last season she was a babysitter, now she's a potential girlfriend. And the explosion at the lunch counter--another good Roy moment, as he saw a dangerous situation and dealt with it. The fact that it gave him the opportunity to put the jerk owner in his place was a bonus. Then of course the place blew up. I even heard the crunch of glass as the squad pulled up--nice touch! And in another example of a victim working with a limited dialogue, the man kept saying "the pain! the pain!" (Sounded a little like Tattoo from Fantasy Island.)

The building where they responded on the comatose boy is the same one with the girdle lady from Peace Pipe. You can easily recognize that church they pass about a block before they get there.

In the final scene Johnny was reading a magazine called Editor and Publisher. I wonder what that's all about? (Note: in Peace Pipe, the book Chet was reading was titled The Problemed Indian. No, that's not a typo on my part, that was the title of the book Chet had, Problemed Indian. Maybe the 'problem' was that the anthropologist was pretentious in his use of words.)

* Nuns-- most of the nuns in my Catholic school were the stereotypical older, knuckle-rapping kind. There *was* one young, pretty nun, Sister Charlene, but in my experience, she was the exception and definitely not the rule.

Edit: Roy's mic-pack is clearly visible under his shirt (middle of his back) in at least one scene at the bus crash. Johnny's is the same, you can even see the wire running up from the pack over his shoulder (when he first gets to the front of the bus).

Edit #2: Watch Roy's hands in the opening scene at the station. From Johnny's POV (facing Roy), Roy's hands are clasped together; when the camera is behind Roy, facing Johnny, he has his hands on his coffee cup.

* * *

Brackett did order an IV, you can hear Johnny open the pack over the biophone, and we see him hang it up on some of the bus wreckage. In fact, Brackett even says "better start a second IV." So one of the boys would have had to accompany the good sister anyway.

Ooh, just thought of something. In the final scene, I believe Roy came into the rec room at the station saying "Good news, Sister Barbara is going to be OK." (And it's sweet that he was so happy about that.) But that was *two days* after the bus crash... did it really take that long for the doctors to feel optimistic about her? Yeah, I know, she was pretty badly injured internally... even if she did manage to still look serene and beautiful and saint-like. I just found the timing a little odd. (Even on his day off, I can definitely see Roy calling Rampart to check on her. He's just that kind of adorable.)

~ ~ ~

How often does the first scene of this show *not* feature either station 51 or at least the paramedics? This ep began at Rampart, which doesn't happen very often.

~ Two episodes in a row with Johnny referencing his background. Except in this one, he says he was raised "on a ranch" instead of a reservation (although he did supposedly learn roping from "my people").

~ So Nurse Sally has a bunch of guys following her around? (Oh wait, that's only true in this *one* episode, because it's handy for the storyline.) And by the way, I think Nurse Ellen was just as pretty as Sally, if not prettier. Actually, I'd give Ellen the edge.

~ Bobby Troup's daughter in yet another episode.

~ So the guy from F-Troop blew up his dive hot dog shack. Did I miss something in that one? Johnny and Roy got him out of the building asap because it was still dangerous in there, and once they set him down Johnny starts putting that sterile cloth over him and Roy gets the biophone. As soon as he contacts Rampart, Roy's giving the guy's vitals. They didn't have a chance to *get* any vitals, all the equipment was still in the squad. Not to mention, I don't know how they could get a BP if his arms were so burned, and probably couldn't get a pulse on his wrist either.

~ Roy claims he doesn't know much about ropes... but as a fireman, I assume he knows more than the average Joe. (Although he didn't look too handy during that knot-tying drill. Sometimes I swear Kevin just skates through stuff his character is supposed to know.)

~ In Peace Pipe I mentioned that we'd see Girdle-girl's building again soon, and *ta-da!*, we saw it today in Saddled. The comatose boy lived in the same building.

~ We see the trestle bridge again in this one too.

~ I didn't mention it in earlier comments, but in the 2nd season the elevator is now in place at Rampart. That space at the end of the hall past the base station was some sort of holding room in the first season, but apparently Rampart's construction is complete and it's now an elevator.

~ I must admit I really like the nun-on-the-bus rescue. It had a lot of good elements: teamwork, additional firefighters (another engine and a snorkel truck), even Chet and Marco got into the act with patching up the kids. And of course there was Sister Barbara. I know I've said this before, but I'm betting that in the 'real incident' this was based on, the nun was probably a pock-marked 60-year-old. Or maybe it wasn't even a nun--could have been a school principal, male or female. But the beautiful young nun was a nice touch. And she had a good connection with both Johnny and Roy. (Love the way she said "Hi, Johnny Gage.") Anyway, I just like the whole thing.

~ The prayer she asked Roy to read is called The Memorare.

~ When Roy was telling Brackett it would be a while yet before they freed the victim, Brackett says "you better start another IV." But that's all he said, he never said what kind of IV. D5W? Saline? Orange juice?

~ Also, while J and R were working with the nun, we'd periodically hear sirens, but I don't know what they were. They sounded like ambulance sirens, but we already saw two ambulances at the scene (Cap requested two of them). And both were still there the next time they showed the road. So I don't know what those sirens were supposed to be.

~ Roy DeSoto and John Gage... angels in blue.(Or... blue angels??)

*   *   *

In at least one episode that I can think of off the top of my head (the super-religious parents who didn't want treatment for their kid, and Brackett called the chaplain to help), the writers made it seem like "religious = nuts," which I didn't like.

I thought it was cute when Sister Barbara asked Roy to read the prayer and he said "I'm not Catholic." Sweet—and funny, as if he was afraid that his not being Catholic would nullify the effect of the prayer, or that his tongue would burn off when he said the words. She only asked you to read the words, Roy, not convert and offer up your first-born. But you could tell that this rescue kind of had an effect on Roy, and that was nice to see. Just as nice was that John was touched as well and respected the connection Sr. Barbara had with Roy.

2.7 Fuzz Lady

I thought I'd get my thoughts down on this episode before I get engrossed in other things.

So... Fuzz Lady. As usual, everyone's dumbfounded at seeing "one of them lady cops you hear tell about." In fact, she was "far out." Pardon my large sighs, but I hate hearing the so-called popular jargon of the day in these shows (my ears were still burning from Adam-12 where someone said "just groove with us." UGH!!).

Anyway, how many times in this show has Roy poured himself a cup of coffee and had Johnny or someone pick it up and drink it?? And we'll never know what he had in the bag he brought in with him. Let's just hope it didn't need to be refrigerated 'cuz they had to bail before he could open it or get a sip of his (replacement) coffee. (Did we all notice that the "real" station 127 was shown when they got the first call? There were some unidentified doors from the apparatus room, and aside from Roy, Johnny, and Cap, the others who ran to the engine must have been the real FFs on duty that day.)

On the Code Blue call at the hospital for the old man, all our 'usual' ED doctors ran to another floor to deal with good ol' Pop. Are they the *only* doctors at Rampart?? Pop was no longer in the ED, so there must have been other doctors on that floor he was on. But no, it's Early and Brackett (and Dixie) to save the day!!

The grandpa in the rocket segment... did we all recognize him? Not only was he "Old Bill" who hung out at the hospital because he was lonely, but he was the husband who brought in his wife and Dixie charmed and consoled him with--what else??--a cup of coffee!

When the "fuzz lady" arrested the thief at Rampart, Johnny was a hoot holding onto the gun, and did you see Roy as he handcuffed the bad guy?? "Excuse me," he said. Too funny!

At the final rescue, when Vince was explaining what had happened with the boat, and Johnny cut the padlock with the bolt cutters, he seemed to have a bit of trouble and when he got it cut, the door kind of flew open and almost knocked into Johnny. I think Vince ad-libbed there and said something like "That was a tough one, wasn't it?" But like the troupers that they were, they kept rolling

More stock footage in this ep... I'll have to get my adult beverage ready and get to the 'drinking game' thread.

* * *

Lastly, I guess the big mystery of this episode is why, after his big date, Johnny needed aspirin for his sore shoulder. My guess is that Fuzz Lady flipped him like she did the perp in the park; either she was demonstrating her skills, or.... Johnny-boy got too fresh. You decide.

~ ~ ~

I'm glad I'm not the only one who didn't care for the Fuzz Lady storyline. (In fact, I'm not gaga about Sharon Gless in either of her guest appearances on this show.) In any case, yeah, Johnny is inconsistent: one season he doesn't like a girl pursuing him, and the next season he does. And this character just wasn't very pleasant to begin with. Come on, Gage, quit basing your opinions of women solely on looks.

Speaking of the female deputy and when the guys first meet her, the call came in definitely at night, as it was full dark as they were driving. But when they got to the park, it looked like it was late afternoon and in the shade. I know, the scene was probably filmed with a filter to try to make it look like night, but imho it didn't work.

Segueing into other things that didn't work... that whole first conversation at the station with Roy and Johnny was one big bag of continuity errors. First Roy pours himself a cup of coffee (and I wonder what was in the bag??). He turns to put the coffee pot back and John walks in and picks up Roy's cup. Seeing this, Roy pours himself *another* cup and sits down at the table. From this point on, you can play "Watch the disappearing cup." Looking at Roy over Johnny's shoulder, we clearly see the coffee cup in front of Roy. But when perspective changes to show us Johnny from over Roy's shoulder, the table in front of Roy is clear--*no coffee cup.* Funny to watch the tennis match of the cup: it's there! it's gone! there! gone!

(Scene goofs, part II) Then the tones go off and we get more bad continuity. For one thing (1): we didn't see or hear anyone else in the dayroom during that conversation, but when the tones go off, the view from the apparatus bay shows a whole bunch of FFs pouring in... from the dayroom. Now, on to (2): Sam times out the call at 0840, but the clock says something very different. And then (3), after jotting down the info, Cap hands it to Roy and then steps back to let the squad go... even though the call was for *Station 51*, including the engine, and in fact we do see the engine roll out along with the squad. Some editor just used the wrong stock footage, or didn't edit the scene carefully enough.

~ The house with the fire and "Pop"... I get the feeling we've seen that house before. Or rather, we will see it again.

~ Grandpa with the rocket is the same actor who played "Old Bill" in an episode, and also a guy named Sam, who brought his wife Martha in and was so worried about losing her.

~ Wasn't the Saturn 1 a rocket of some sort? And it's also a piece of medical equipment at Rampart. Just like a Bird ventilator isn't really a bird ventilator.

~ After helping the Do-It-All Doctors with installing the pacemaker in Pop, Dixie put her nurse's cap back on... without any hairpins. Somehow I think that defies the laws of physics.

~ Is this the first time we see friction between Morton and the paramedics? It only pops up occasionally when required for script purposes; otherwise they all get along great.

~ And yeah, the arrest in the parking garage at Rampart was pretty eye-rolling. Johnny's reluctantly holding a loaded weapon (worse, he's sort of waving it around), and Roy begs the perp's pardon before cuffing him. That has to be the politest police restraint in history. (And the most unbelievable, all the way around.)

~ For the final rescue, the guy stuck on the crane, I too noticed that Cap said stokes when he meant gurney. But did anyone else notice all the stokes that were literally hanging around that pier? No wonder he got confused and said the wrong thing. I saw at least two separate ones, I wonder why they were there?

2.8 Trainee

I noticed the canteen in the squad too, and thought, "huh"??
It sort of makes sense that they'd have one, especially for
tough rescues or fires or whatever, but we've never seen it
before, I don't think, so it just seemed to come from out of
the blue.

Every now and then when the guys arrive on a call, a victim
or family member will say "I called our family doctor, etc."
First of all, how long would it take the doctor to be available,
and would he (most likely a he) make a house call? We even
heard about the family doctor in the episode Problem, when
the car engine fell on the guy. Really, even if the guy had
gotten to Rampart as soon as the jerky doctor wanted, what
would he be able to do?? The family doctor is usually a GP-
-how well equipped would he be to deal with multiple
internal injuries?

I had to chuckle at the scene in the washroom at the station,
with Johnny and Marlowe, and then Roy when he came in...
they kept saying how he "fouled up." Yeah, like *that's* the
word they'd use in real life!! You'd think they could at least
say "screwed up"... I don't think it was considered 'vulgar'
back in the day, was it??

And I agree about Marlowe's situation... on one hand, it had
been years since he returned from Vietnam (almost the *only*
reference to the 'war' that this show ever made), so you'd
think he would have adjusted pretty well, since even Roy
said he was a good, smart firefighter. On the other hand, his
paramedic training might have brought his 'god complex'
back to the fore. On the third hand (wait, what?) I have
trouble believing that after five years he has trouble grasping

the concept of "chain of command," especially since those years were spent in the fire service, which is all about chain of command. But you're right that he could have really used some support from other vets... in 1973 LA must have been crawling with them, and there had to be others in the LACoFD. Heck, even Roy had been in the Army, which we *never* hear about except for maybe two very quick references. Speaking of feeling sorry for Marlowe.... if this particular storyline was 'real' and based on a real occurrence in the FD, can you imagine how the real-life Marlowe must have felt when this episode aired?? Hopefully the story was changed and exaggerated for TV.

It was funny to watch Chet's face while Marlowe was sounding off to him about John and Roy. When Marlowe said "I've seen them, I've watched them play it safe," I wish Chet had spoken up for them, maybe saying "I've seen them work, too, and if my sister or my mother was ever in an accident, Gage and DeSoto are the ones I'd want to get her out." It would have been a nice touch to have Chet clearly and unequivocally put himself on Team R-and-J.

Speaking of Johnny... he got quite a workout in this episode, didn't he? First he chases a thief (and gets all sweaty in the process, not to mention injured), then he falls down a cliff, and he even runs after the car-wash guy. No wonder he was able to stay so skinny!

By the way, in the carwash scene, at one point or another you can see the mic-packs on all three guys, under their shirts (on their backs).

Also (yeah, I know this is long, but I have to type it before I forget it), was it just me or was this ep a little like watching a ping-pong game? In the first scene, Roy and Johnny think the trainee's "gonna work out fine." In the next scene they're butting heads, big time. Then the very next scene is days later and they not only think he's going to work out fine, but they're joking about having him as a partner. A minute later the tones sound, they go out on a call, and they're butting heads again, and 10 minutes later Johnny's saying Marlowe isn't going to work out. Their attitudes changed so often, I thought I was going to get whiplash.

But of course, Roy called it from the get-go (he's "overtrained"), and it's Roy who delivers the big dressing-down. Good speech, Roy!

* * *

I thought it was an interesting detail (and realistic) that once the chopper dropped the stokes, Roy motioned for it to move off, and the chopper swung out over the water. A minor detail, perhaps, but again, realistic, as there's no way they could deal with the victim with the rotors churning above them.

I wondered why Johnny didn't take the biophone with him when he went "topside." He said the phone still worked, and they wouldn't have needed LA to relay the info. Plus, it would have been one less piece of equipment for Roy and Marlowe to pack up and take with them. **BUT....** since the phone did still work after the tumble down the cliff, I guess he left it for Roy to take and communicate with Rampart from the chopper while en route. (Sort of answered my own question, I guess....)

An interesting point about the different ways Roy and Johnny try to get through to Marlowe. Sort of mirrors their personalities in a way-- one hot-tempered and outspoken (or, as you say, "blunt"), the other analytical and circumspect, but definitely no less intense.

~ ~ ~

Okay, this is a heavy episode, sort of an "issues" episode, as it's the first time we see the guys deal with a paramedic trainee. It's also sort of a PSA episode, which educates viewers on how the paramedic program worked during those early years in LA County.

In the previous discussion of this one, I mentioned that I felt like I got whiplash, trying to keep up with John and Roy's opinions of Ed Marlowe. On their very first day, on the cliff, Roy had to get in his face and practically threatened to wash him out on their first 'real' rescue. Then suddenly it's two weeks later or so (no clear segue to tell us that), and both paramedics are suddenly high on Marlowe and joking about partnering up with him, at which point the tones sound and off they go on another run. A scant hour later Johnny's ready to wash his hands of Marlowe for good, and Roy is close. So first they're happy with Ed, then they're not, then they are again, but suddenly they're not. The writing could have been more consistent on this matter—or at least explained the time frame.

In the beginning (chasing the purse-snatcher), it was almost like watching an episode of Adam-12: the light-haired veteran stays with the crime victim while the younger dark-haired partner goes in foot pursuit. And I'm sure we all noticed the funky canteen they used after the chase. Nowadays that would be plastic water bottles or one big keg-type container like sports teams use. (Also, I thought it was odd that the dispatcher inquired about their status and then said "call this office your next stop." Wonder what that was all about, I don't think I've heard that before, a request for them to call dispatch.) Also, it was weird that the deputy brought Marlowe back, and Marlow was in the *back* seat. Was the perp in the front seat? Or was it another deputy? Maybe another car picked up the perp? I dunno.

The call to the guy who fell off the cliff... I wonder why the dispatch said "you will be responding alone." Don't believe I've ever heard that before, either.

Johnny's slide and tumble down that embankment looked totally real.

When the squad pulled up to the house with the OD woman, that poor husband was telling his life story to all of them, and first one paramedic, then a second, and finally the last one (Roy) just walked away from him without answering. Roy could at least have answered when the guy said "Did I do the right thing?" I felt bad that nobody even acknowledged the poor guy.

By the way, when the call came for the OD, and Roy and Johnny were in the office joking about partnering with Marlowe, the clock in the office had the 'right' time that matched the call, but the one in the apparatus bay was completely different.

I always have to laugh when I see Brackett or someone insert an esophageal airway... always looks fake (when they do show it, that is, as they usually don't). And it looks fake for a reason.

The confrontation at the station of Johnny and Marlowe, and then Roy and Marlowe, is always good to watch. It's actually a pretty intense scene, imho. Even though I do have to chuckle a little when I hear them talk about "fouling up." Yeah, because *that's* how firefighters talk. Also, when Roy called Ed a "dangerous character"... I just find that so cute and amusing for some reason.

Lastly, at the car wash, what the heck kind of car (?) was that vehicle where Marlowe caught up with the victim? Was that an early version of the El Camino? Whatever it was, I thought it was kind of ugly.

2.9 Women

So a number of episodes were all written by the same writer who wrote this episode? Off the top of my head I can't recall if any of them are some of the "offending" episodes we've mentioned. I think one was Dinner Date, when Roy was trying to fix John up with Joanne's friend or something. I can't recall which episode it is where Johnny lists all the nurses at Rampart, how many were single, how many were "too tall," how many were "too old," "too fat," etc. That was another prize conversation.

I agree, this episode was painful to listen to. Do these writers know how to create any guest characters who aren't extreme in some way? No Goldilocks here.... they're all *too* abrasive, or *too* meek, *too* opinionated, or *too* something else. None are "just right."

I actually wrote a review of this episode elsewhere. Without rehashing what I wrote there, here are a few other tidbits I noticed this time around.

~ Not only do we get to see the engine roll out first, in front of the squad, but we also get to see our favorite trestle bridge. (And there's a RR identifier sign next to the tracks, that has '4' on it. Not that that will help finding it on Google Earth.)

~ Why are parents always depicted as being so clueless? "My child never does drugs. My kid is a good boy." Etc. And the other extreme was the little boy's mother, the hemlock kid's mother. She didn't seem upset or hysterical, when she was in the treatment room she almost seemed frustrated, as if she was annoyed with the doctors and with the kid. At first I thought she was a babysitter, as she seemed so detached and unemotional.

~ This episode had Dick Van Patten (from Grateful) and also "Millie Helper," the actress from the Dick Van Dyke show. Hmm, I wonder if she has a 'thing' for actors named Dick Van Something.

~ Re Christy... was it just me or did it seem like, even for 1972, her camera didn't seem like something a professional would use? She looked like a nosy tourist. Also, during her little rant in the rec room, I was sort of waiting for (or *hoping* for) Roy to do his thing and put her in her place. Too bad he didn't. He's good at that sort of thing, but maybe he was all worn out from doing it to Ed Marlowe just the week before.

~ Since when do the paramedics "need" the victim's name before contacting Rampart? Every now and then they give the name over the biophone, as if it's going to make a difference to Dr. Early if the guy's name is Joe Jones or Bill Smith. Nothing but a plot device, supposedly "necessary" when it fits the script.

~ Oh, yeah, I think we've noticed a few other stock scenes when "real" members of Station 127/51 are shown running to the engine. In this episode, when they were rolling out for the exploding building, the camera is on the back of the engine, and those "real" FFs must have been in the engine, because those guys in the jump seats were *not* Chet and Marco. For the most part they kept their heads down so we mainly saw their helmets, but we did get brief glimpses of their faces, so you could tell they weren't "our" station 51 guys.

*   *   *

Oh yes, the whole "girls can work, but only until they get married" notion. Back in the '40s I believe they were called "career girls." They were the young women who went to secretarial school and got jobs, probably (stereotypically) hoping to meet the boss's son and get married, at which time they'd 'get to' quit working. A woman's identity was always connected to the men in her life (first the father, and then the husband), and working at a paying job was something she wasn't expected to do unless she had to, to support herself. And yes, the most common (and acceptable) professions for women were nurses, secretaries, or teachers.

Funny how women were expected to move from their father's house to their husband's, and transfer their identity from "Mr. Smith's daughter" to "Mr. Jones' wife." On Adam-12, and even sometimes on Emergency (early to mid '70s), women will identify themselves as "I'm Mrs. Robert Johnson"... as if their own first name is irrelevant and unnecessary. These days, who does that?? Hopefully, nobody.

I guess the John Gage of 1972 wouldn't care for my ideas and would call me a "women's libber." Luckily "women's lib" is no longer an active movement, as such great strides have been made in 40 years that we don't think about it as much. Not that all equality issues have been solved, by any stretch of the imagination; but in general young girls and boys no longer have rigid expectations of what is 'women's work' or 'a man's job,' at least not nearly as much as back then.

~ ~ ~

~ When leaving on first call, Johnny was in a bit of a snit when he got in the squad next to Christy, and when Cap handed Roy the sheet with the address, Johnny was busy

93

getting his helmet set, so Roy just dropped the paper in his lap. I just thought that was kinda cute.

~ At the accident scene, the deputy had already requested the power be cut to those lines, but since they couldn't wait for that, Cap had Marco and Chet cut the actual lines. So why then did he ask again how long it would be until the power was cut? Not sure if that made sense.

~ Yes, at Rampart we have a classic case of SPS-- Stupid Parent Syndrome. Drugs? Not *my* kid! Booze? No way, I would know! Teen sex? He/she is a good kid, nothing like that could *ever* happen!... he said as his OD'ing pregnant daughter was wheeled in. *eye-roll* (Yeah, the girl in the show wasn't pregnant--that we know of--but you get the point.)

~ I too saw the irony in Christy checking her face in the mirror and cleaning up before going in to the rescue. Pot, meet kettle. And that wife really was a piece of work. What a shrew! Great irony there as well, Miss Christy Todd, but I bet you didn't notice *that*.

~ Back at the station, I thought it was kinda amusing, Roy's choice of word when talking to the other guys, words which today would (or could) have a whole different meaning. He said "If you'd stop riding her, she might write something nice." Haha, if Johnny *did* "ride her," she might write something better. (Sorry, that was a bit crass, I guess.)

~ At the final explosion rescue, I liked all the sawdust that was falling everywhere, I thought that was a nice touch. But even though Station 51 was the first company at the scene, I heard all the "big crowd" sound effects, of firefighters shouting and saying the same things on a loop.

~ And I couldn't agree more about the random little girl trapped in the building. Whiskey tango foxtrot?? That was totally bogus and gratuitous and just a reason to have Johnny somehow get trapped inside. And when Roy came in and found him, he left his flashlight, so that's another piece of LACoFD equipment that got left behind.

~ Final scene: not sure why Roy needs to shave at the station... at the start of his shift. I can maybe see the guys sticking around once their shift is over and showering/shaving before they go home, but why shave upon arrival? Makes no sense. And I had to chuckle at Johnny's use of the phrase *groove on*. "She grooves on hostility."

~ Speaking of that, I also call bogus on Johnny pretending his 'hostility' was part of some grand plan. We all know that John Gage isn't that good of an actor (he can't play poker, after all). His rants about Christy when she wasn't around are proof that he really did dislike her.

Ugh. Sorry, I have to stop now. I dislike the whole Christy thing. But oddly enough, for a change I do like the stories that take place at Rampart in this one. Go figure.

~ ~ ~

Review of this episode, printed elsewhere:

This episode, in my opinion, has not stood the test of time, as the main conflict in it is no longer an issue today, and something that anyone under the age of 30 wouldn't be able to identify with. Regardless, it at least gives food for thought.

The journalist assigned to ride with Squad 51 is a woman--a young, very attractive woman (Christy). Of course, Gage finds her charming... until she opens her mouth and challenges and questions everything that the paramedics--and even the firefighters--do. "I could have done that.

Women can do that too," is her refrain. Her reverse chauvinism is off- putting and grating.

To me, the biggest failing of this episode is the lack of follow-up, and the fact that the storyline didn't get thoroughly explained. For one thing, I want to know what Dixie had to say to Christy. After the arrogant journalist takes Brackett to task for his perceived attitude of male superiority (in his own department, no less!), Dixie suggests the two women have a cup of coffee. And personally, I want to know what they talked about! Dixie is a very confident woman; she's surrounded by headstrong men on a daily basis, and not only does *she* not feel they're superior to her, the men themselves don't think that either. If anyone could, Dixie might have been able to give Christy a better perspective of the people she was supposed to be writing about (paramedics, firefighters, doctors), all of whom just happen to be men. Secondly, it was commented on more than once that whatever article this woman writes could have an impact on the public's opinion of the paramedic program (and firefighting in general), but not once do we hear what she actually ends up writing about for her article. Was it fair? Complimentary? Glowing, even? At the building explosion site, after Roy helps Johnny escape just before it blows, viewers are led to believe that she might be 'seeing the light' about firefighters and how they're willing to brave imminent danger to help others as well as 'one of their own,' and yet, we don't get to find out if that's true since, again, we don't know what she finally wrote. I suppose firefighting can be a real "boy's club;" it's still dominated by men and I'm sure a fire station can probably have an atmosphere like a sports locker room, but still, this woman was judging every firefighter by whatever preconceptions she had, whether true or not, without giving them the benefit of the doubt. (Plus, did anyone else think it odd? Here she is a journalist, and she's five feet away from a man who's been sought by the police for blowing up buildings... and she didn't even *try* to talk to him??? Not much of a journalist, imho!)

Lastly, the BIG mystery is... how did Johnny get a date with her? They had been at daggers drawn for the whole time she was with Station 51, and most of that time he couldn't stand to be in the same room with her. So what happened? Did he ask her out in spite of his dislike of her? Did she ask *him* out? Obviously any explanation that Johnny Gage gives about women should be taken with a grain (or shaker) of salt, so how did that *really* come to pass?? Inquiring minds do want to know!!

2.10 Dinner Date

Ah, Dinner Date. Yes, one of the offending episodes from the wonderful writers who don't hesitate to call any woman a "dog" if she didn't look like Cheryl Tiegs (pulling a name from back in the day). By the way, I wonder if that applies to the wife/sister/daughter/niece of the guy who wrote that crap storyline. Ah well, I'll get back to that.

I too thought the little bicyclist didn't look anywhere near ten, much less over that age. And yeah, even after the mother sent him home (across the street without even looking), she hung around to be nosy with the other girl. .. And did we all recognize the epileptic woman? She was the same actress who played the "lady paramedic" in San Francisco in the two E! movies. Guess she loved what she saw in LA and decided to become one in SF. Did anyone else get jealous, er, notice how Roy put his arm around her somewhat protectively? And people wonder why the chicks dig DeSoto!!

Speaking of, it was a little heartbreaking to see Melissa Gilbert cry for her daddy and Roy give her a big hug like that. He's good at that sort of thing, apparently. And, okay, ugh! I just watched part of a video on YouTube about "jugular stick." Which is exactly what it sounds like, they "stick" the needle in the jugular. (Silly, me, I thought the 'stick' was a noun, a description of a different piece of equipment, rather than a verb, referring to where the IV is inserted.)

Meanwhile, it was "Drug Awareness Week" at the hospital. Luckily we had no PIDs (Parents in Denial) like we had in yesterday's episode (Women). This time the mother knew and suspected, so good for her and good for the writer for getting *that* right, at least.

Yeah, about the "very obese" car victim... I kind of always feel bad for the actors who are hired for a job and told "you're going to be picked on for being fat," or "your character is considered very ugly," etc. I know, I know, these things don't come out of the blue, and actors know what they look like and know what to expect from certain roles, but still.

How about the multiple gunshot victim who only had a little bit of blood on his shoulder? I've bled more than that when I cut my leg shaving.

Anyone notice that we didn't see the "other guys" until the last sequence? Every now and then we'll see only ONE of the station guys (usually Chet, sometimes Cap), until they all appear at a rescue later in the episode.

Dr. Early made a point to say "if a parent is available for permission, administer such-and-such IV" to the girl in the pool, but Johnny never actually asked the mother for permission. I guess he thought it was implied. Also, here's another detail that's small and very specific and probably gets missed by 90% of people who watch the show, but I love it when the guys (and it's usually Roy) puts pieces of tape on his leg in preparation for administering an IV. We don't often see him actually use the tape on the patient, but it's there, it's an added detail that makes the scene look real. (And I wonder why it is always Roy... maybe he and Johnny flipped a coin and decided that Roy has to be the one to tape up his pants.)

Now back to the dinner date and the aftermath thereof.... in a way the story reminded me of a similar conversation from an episode of Adam-12. Reed (the married one) invited Pete to dinner to meet his wife's friend. Tired of all the set-ups that don't go well, Pete wasn't enthused and weaseled out of it. (There may have been a similar conversation about wondering what the woman looked like, I don't recall; but now I'm curious so I might have to look for it.) Anyway, Reed happens to mention that the girl is "a model" and of course Pete's ears perk up and suddenly "hey, I might be able to make it to dinner after all." Typical man!! What would be worse, to spend three hours with a beautiful woman who can't hold a conversation, or three hours with a "plain Jane" who is interesting and smart and funny??

> Oh, that shirt on Johnny in the last scene! I bet if you stared at it long enough, you'd see that pattern on everything you looked at.

I'm sorry, did you say something about that scene? My attention was on Roy's pretty white shirt and his pretty blue eyes....

* * *

I totally agree about Johnny's Best Moments. When he's ranting about computers taking over the world, or his paycheck being held out from him... meh, pass. But when he's ranting about trainee paramedics who are endangering patients, or doctors/interns who question the paramedics' judgements in the field..... bring it on, baby!!

And I totally agree, sometimes (when his hair isn't out of control) John Gage is just plain...*pretty*. I've seen screen caps of him where he looks like he could be a Michelangelo sculpture; a veritable feast for the eyes. And yet... I remain unaffected; what can I say, I'm contrary like that. Again, I don't go for the obvious, don't fall for the flash. (Just like with Adam-12: Reed is the classically handsome one, and I recognize and appreciate his dark good looks, but it's not for me. Of the two, Malloy might not catch the eye right away, but when you look twice you realize he's the total package.) And the way the writers wrote Johnny sort of split his character in two, with the sane, serious, rational side on the one hand, and the extreme goofiness and shallowness on the other hand; makes my head spin.

I also agree about Johnny trying to be "Joe Cool." I think most of the reason he struck out with women was because he just plain tried too hard. Always working an angle to try to impress. That might get a guy noticed, but most likely not anything beyond that. Slow your roll, Gage!

No, I didn't have any preference (i.e., crush) when I was young (I can't even say for sure how often I watched the show, back in the day) but as an adult, I think I'd probably give Joanne a run for her money when it comes to the deceptively mild-mannered Roy DeSoto. Bad hair days notwithstanding, he had the charm and personality that's more attractive in the long run. (And the eyes-- let's not forget the eyes....) Besides, have you seen him with his shirt off? Roy kind of reminds me of Ned Flanders from The Simpsons... you see him in normal clothes and he looks one way, but see him without his shirt and it's a *whole* different ballgame!! (I'm thinking in particular of a picture of Kevin from a TV gig he did toward the end of Emergency, where he's on a beach.... oh, mama!!)

~ ~ ~

Today's lesson, kids, is this: booze and drugs--just say no! Seriously, that was the theme of this episode. And I have to wonder if Bobby and Julie needed a bunch of takes to get through their coffee-room scene with a straight face, since they were probably quite familiar with the topic from their nightclub days.

Anyhoo, moving right along....

~ The kid who wasn't hit by a car: who remembers spider bikes?? With the requisite banana seat, of course. And did we all notice the boy's mom who not only ran across the street with barely a glance at traffic (and pretty much told her son to do the same), but also, she threatened that he better do it before she decided to "get a switch." My, how times have changed!

~ The young woman who was epileptic, did she look familiar to anyone? She would go on to play the paramedic in San Francisco... the one married to the absent-minded professor. In that one movie she looked like she might have had an eye for Roy, during that conversation they had at the hospital.

~ Here it is in season two and Rampart is still using some glass bottles for IVs.

~ We saw more of the squad in this one episode than we normally see in five or six, particularly in the scene when Roy brought up the suggestion of the dinner date. Johnny was putting stuff into that compartment that's directly behind the cab (*not* the one where they keep drug box, biophone, etc.); I thought that's where he keeps his turnout coat, but it wasn't in there.

~ Not sure if I've ever mentioned this before (and maybe it belongs in Random Musings and Observations), but every time they send an EKG, that machine at Rampart that prints out the strip always reminds me of the sounds that the computers make on the original Star Trek. Since I'm not a big fan of Star Trek TOS, this drives me nuts.

~ Okay, in case the heavy-handed PSA elements of this episode weren't enough, then the writer added a funny bit of irony. The teen girl who'd been given the tainted drugs, her mother said "we keep alcohol in the house, like everyone does," and later after she leaves the treatment room, what does she do but pop a few pills herself. She already told Brackett she uses tranquilizers, so between that and the booze... is it any wonder her daughter got the wrong idea?? (I'll stop now, I don't need to hop onto *that* particular train of thought.)

~ The man with the pacemaker they had to pull out of his car: I wonder how that guy would be described today. "Very obese"? He was certainly overweight and out of shape but I'm not sure the "very" was warranted. And I hate to say it, but there are cops and paramedics today who look like that guy did if not worse.

~ Did anyone see Cap trip as he first approached the car? He almost lost his helmet.

~ Speaking of the EKG making that computerized, futuristic noise, when the guys sent the pacemaker man's strip, the machine made the Star Trek noise. Except when Brackett communicated back to Roy. The machine was still pushing out the strip, but the noise miraculously went away as soon as Brackett pushed the button on the phone to talk to the paramedics. (And no, I don't think the equipment is set up that way... that's just what the producers did so we could hear Brackett talk.)

~ Not to laugh at Lockjaw Guy, but I did have to roll my eyes a little. Joe Early told the nurse to "take him and admit him to ICU." Yeah, it's just that simple: you don't need any paperwork, no forms signed by any other doctor with instructions, just wheel him on up there and say, "Hey, here's a guy for you from Dr. Early. He's all yours now."

~ I can't ignore the title of this episode, and the (once again) demeaning way the writers had Johnny talk about girls/women. He referred to one as a dog and then was ready to judge this new one by how much she weighed. Bad writers--bad, bad writers! By the way, when Roy first asked Johnny what he was doing that night, Johnny said "oh, I dunno, driving up to Santa Barbara I guess," or something like that. Was going to Santa Barbara the equivalent of hanging out at the mall or whatever it is that people do when they don't have any other plans? It sounded weird to me.

2.11 Musical Mania

Wow, two lockjaw cases in as many episodes?? I do remember hearing about it when I was a kid, so I guess it happened often enough that the writers felt the need to do a PSA about it. And this episode also has another PID-- Parent in Denial of child's drug use. This one ended tragically, although it brought us a nice moment of reflection from John and Roy. "My parents weren't that indifferent." And thank heavens for that!

The actor who played Boyd in this episode was also in today's ep of Adam-12. Funky, huh?? Speaking of, I hate to say it but I don't care for how the writers characterized the Boyds. They were poor and a little naive, so of course they had to be from some backwoods state. I mean, Piney Grove, or wherever they came from, could have been in Minnesota, or New York, or Indiana, right??

In the treatment room with the OD girl, Johnny presented his cute butt toward the camera and he took something out of his pocket. I noticed a cord or something coming out of his pocket which looked like the thin earbud cords for an iPod, and the thing he took out of his back pocket was about the size and shape of an iPod. But I didn't recognize what it was. Also, right after that, after he hung some stuff on the pole, Johnny kind of had to move Morton's arm out of the way so he could get by. It was sort of cute.

Should we assign Brackett to clean the latrine in punishment? Dixie said something about setting up one of the rooms (I think) and he said "Good girl." It's not terribly offensive, but still, cringeworthy at the very least.

Also, why doesn't Dr. Early have an office? Brackett is the only one who does. In the first episode or the pilot or something, I think the two of them shared that office (two desks), but eventually it became Brackett's office.

In the scene with Johnny playing the bagpipes, I wonder what book Roy was reading? And we got a reference to Chet studying for the engineer exam. In a later scene, how exciting is it to sit around watching two people play chess?? That's not how I'd spend my free time. I mean, they do have a television, don't they?

Strange question... has anyone noticed the dangerous "decapitation corner" at Rampart? When people walk in from the Emergency entrance and turn onto the main corridor, there are some overhead cabinets there on the corner that are potentially dangerous. In an early episode (can't remember which one) Roy puts his hand up as he passes, to shield himself from the sharp corner at the bottom. Now, in this episode, I see they parked some big-a$$ piece of equipment there, probably so nobody inadvertently smacks into it.

~ ~ ~

In a couple small ways, this episode was somewhat of a continuation of yesterday's themes: the evils of drugs, an Egyptian parent (who lived in de-Nile), a victim who's too heavy (fat) for his own good, and even another case of lockjaw. Yes, quite a coincidence. But that's really neither here nor there.

~ One thing I wondered (and forgive me if this has been addressed before)... on Adam-12 I think I heard that many of the addresses used in the show are purposely incorrect so that people/onlookers don't go to the locations, and I can't remember if the same thing was done on Emergency! But I wondered if all the locations/addresses used on the show were real.

~ So this was the 2nd ep in a row with tetanus, better known as lockjaw. And did we all recognize Roy's "wife" as the man's daughter? I confess that the first time or two I saw this ep I didn't realize that was the same actress, and only learned it when I heard it elsewhere.

~ Was it weird that Brackett told Dixie "Good girl"? I know times were different then, but still..."girl"?? Also, I can't believe Dixie didn't have a few words for Nurse Nippy at the check-in desk. Not only did said nurse ignore Dixie and the family she was with, but she was pretty rude and dismissive to Boyd. Also, the mom told Dr. Early that the kid was eating the paint because he was teething... but he was *four years old.* My memory may be rusty, but I'm pretty sure that four-year-olds are done with teething by a year or two. Lastly, once again the writers of this show decided that when it comes to non-Hollywood people, "country = ignorant." Or maybe it's "ignorant = country." Just like yesterday, I want to smack the writers on the nose with a rolled-up newspaper.

~ Boy, I heard some squealing brakes when the squad arrived at the scene of the ice-cream truck. I think someone mentioned that previously in other episodes, and here it was. Also, the deputies said they didn't know where the driver was. Um, really??? They'd been there for 10 minutes and didn't see the driver's legs sticking out of the friggin' window?? Not very observant law enforcement officers, are they??

~ The OD teen girl: good rescue. By the way, does anyone else remember playing or having recess on concrete? Those girls were having gym class (volleyball) on the roof of a building. Also, in the treatment room at the hospital, I noticed again that Johnny moved Morton's arm so he could get by. It was kind of cute.

~ After the clueless mom (I actually felt sorry for her, I have to admit) when Roy and Johnny were driving from Rampart they started talking about kids and parents who care, etc. It's middle of the day, bright sunlight, and we see them pass the granary in that commercial, built-up area. But when the camera moves inside the cab and they're talking, the scenery is suddenly much more rural with trees and fields, etc., and looking out Roy's window, it's dusk (or at least overcast) outside. Then, suddenly when the call comes in and the squad speeds away, it's full sun again and they're once again in a commercial area.

~ The guy in the glider—wouldn't it have been easier for him to get out if he unhooked his chute or backpack or whatever it was on his back?

~ Anyone ever notice how Bobby Troup looks down at his hands and rubs one hand against the other when he's speaking or thinking about things?

~ At the station, in the scene when Chet confronts Johnny about his "musical mania," it's no coincidence that Roy says they have "tons" of ice cream products in the freezer. (Wonder how they got it there from the accident site?)But what's funny is that when he tried to eat one, the stick came out of the ice cream in Roy's hand--I wonder if that was supposed to happen??

~ I also like the final rescue. Once again we see a house precariously built over a steep drop-off, and of course someone got stuck underneath when the house decided to follow the laws of gravity. But one thing I couldn't believe was that Johnny went down under the house *without his helmet*. To me that situation seems to be the very definition of why and when a helmet is required. And yet... Gage was bareheaded. Also, they left the Porta-Power down there. Add that to the list of Lost Equipment.

2.12 Helpful

So about Dr. Varner.... As a person (and a doctor) she was fine, but.... I don't like the one-hit-wonder storyline about her. Classic example of someone who's supposedly a 'regular' (even if she is apparently new), and yet we've never heard of her before, and never see her again. Can you say "plot device"?? After Dixie corrected her on the MS call, Dixie kind of behaved as if she had an attitude, but she said "no problem, we're cool," etc. I thought she was kind of sending mixed signals.

When Roy was commiserating with Boot about Johnny giving advice, I saw Boot drool. I hope the guys cleaned it up.

In this ep there was a supposed gang fight, and Rampart was expecting a crowd. Every now and then (like in this instance), we see an ambulance bring in patients, with no paramedics in sight. Did they just do the old "scoop and run" thing, like they did before the paramedic program? I don't think the ambulance attendants can do anything except administer oxygen and put on bandages, like they did with the gang fight guy.

Brackett's clothes.... was that an assault on the senses or what??? Wide-striped tie, paisley-patterned shirt, and narrow-striped pants.

Once again, we see Roy getting dressed in the locker room. (Not that I'm complaining, mind you.) But watching that scene was funny, as he used the "zzzzip" of his pants as sort of an exclamation point to his statement.

Did we all like the express time-lapse during that last rescue, of the kids in the water system? When they got the call and rolled out of the station, it was sunny, looked like about noon, based on shadows. The time of the call was "eight thirty-two," which meant morning. ?!?! But as they were driving, it looked like dusk. And by the time they got to the ugly back-lot set, it was full dark. Go figure!!

Oh, and rack up another lost helmet for Johnny. He had it on when he picked up the lost kid, but when he got up after falling in the water, he didn't have it. Whoops, dock that boy's pay!

* * *

I agree it was nice to see a smart, capable woman doctor. And *(hallelujah!)* nobody made any issue of her being a woman! There was no mistrust of her ability, no snide remarks about her choice of career. Thank heavens the writer did right by the character!!!

(Although.... past episodes have planted the seed of doubt. If she hadn't been from a foreign country, if she'd been an American citizen from Peoria or Tallahassee or Santa Barbara (and she had some other dramatic story for working three jobs), I wonder if the writers would have been as generous, or if they would have given us some "Chet" remarks, or "Ed Wells" attitude. (From Adam-12.)

* * *

And yes, Johnny has a good heart, he just wanted to help his "best friend." Although I do think calling Joanne with Stoker's recipe was *not* the best move. Just because it happened to work out doesn't mean it was right.

~ ~ ~

Ah, Dr. Varner... not one of the better Rampart-based storylines, imho. Again, we've never heard of her before, never hear of her again. Would it kill these powers that be to maybe show the character at least *once* before featuring someone everyone supposedly knows?? (Although John and Roy didn't seem to know her either.) And good point about Dixie being pretty much out of character, but then, she's had a few of those uncharacteristic moments over the past number of episodes.

~ Ha, good point about the fact that patients magically can't hear the doctors when they step three feet away, accusing them of psychosomatic behavior, etc.

~ I thought the FF usual shifts were 1 day on, 2 days off? That would mean a 24-hour shift, not 48. Unless I missed something.... (I guess it varies.)

~ In the first scene, when Johnny displays uncharacteristic perception about Roy's mood, I noticed voices--talk and even laughter--in the background. It actually sounded pleasantly realistic, as if Cap and the other guys were in the dayroom or the office or wherever. Hearing it today made me realize we usually *don't* hear it any other time.

~ Another reference to a boulevard stop. I think I know what they mean, but to me it's annoying as the writers seem to assume that everyone is familiar with the term (and I never was while growing up).

~ Speaking of random doctors, when Johnny called in from that first accident, we see the base station at Rampart and there's some guy (doctor? intern?) standing at the desk. He makes a move toward the radio, as if to answer it, but steps back to the desk as Dixie hurries over. We've never seen that before, I don't think.

~ Cap was cooking. And later Roy was chopping some stuff up for *his* turn as chef. But we only *hear* about Stoker's spaghetti... we didn't get to see it.

~ I thought it was funny when Roy and John arrived at that one scene, and Johnny stopped and looked down, asking, "Is there a dog on the roof?" The way he said it was cute, as if saying "Am I going crazy or is that really there?"

~ Ever notice that there don't seem to be too many well-adjusted couples on this show? The ones we see (on rescues or at Rampart) are almost always one of the following: 1) shrew of a wife and either wimpy husband or 'regular' husband, or 2) domineering (or jerky) husband and meek, submissive wife. I wonder if that's somehow related to the horrible (and very dated) portrayal of women on this show?

~ Don't you just love Dixie's hair when she lets it down? I forgot it was *that* long, but it was beautiful.

~ I had to laugh at the scene at the station when Roy's getting his uniform on and Johnny arrives in the locker room. Roy is pi$$ed that Johnny called Joanne and gave her Stoker's recipe, and Johnny said she was very nice about it. "She was being polite," Roy said in irritation, "you should have been there for the fireworks after she hung up." And after he said that, he sort of 'punctuated' it by zipping up his pants. Not sure if the sound was dubbed, but you could definitely hear it, and even Johnny noticed it and looked down.

~ Either they got the timeline screwed up and the kids-in-storm-drain rescue took place in the evening, or it got unusually scary-dark during that thunderstorm. Because it seemed to be daylight when they left the station, but full dark by the time they arrived at the scene, and it stayed full dark throughout.

~ When they found the two boys, was one of them supposed to be unconscious? I did notice his fingers moving as if he was picking at the concrete, but otherwise I believe he was *supposed* to be unconscious, especially since he didn't move or react when the paramedics got to them. So what does Johnny do? He drops the unconscious kid into the water! I have to say it was pretty bush-league of Gage not to be more careful; he walked right into that heavy stream of water because he wasn't paying attention to his surroundings. And

I have no idea why he fell again later, at the bottom of the stairs. Didn't he eat his Wheaties that morning???

~ I guess Marco and Chet walked in the rain back to where the engine was... they disappeared once Roy got topside. (And yuck, the inside of the squad must've gotten totally soaked with Roy, Johnny, and the two kids in there.)

~ When the squad leaves Rampart for the last time, after this rescue, we see a very tight and unusual view of the two guys inside the cab. There is no passing scenery, no long-shot of the squad driving away, etc. I think it's because it was supposedly still raining, and the show didn't have any stock footage of the squad driving in the rain. Therefore they couldn't show the outside but had to keep the camera focused on the two guys. At least, that's my theory.

2.13 Drivers

Yes, klepto Johnny, caught in the act! My current theory is that the item was something of Randy's that got put or left on that set, and he simply just 'retrieved' it while filming the scene. But who knows???

This is the second time in a couple of days I've heard reference to a "boulevard stop." (Not necessarily both on this show, though.)

They didn't do an IV for the football player, and yet Johnny rode in with him to Rampart. I thought they mainly did that when they administered some medications.

Does anyone else flinch when we hear calls from other squads to Rampart? They always sound so... sterile. No background noise, no sirens, no off-camera exchanges, or "um" or "uh," which normal people do in real, fluid situations. Instead, they sound like exactly what they are: actors reading from a script in a nice, quiet room. For a show that valued realism, that aspect of 'fail' is pretty blatant.

During the football player scene and the boy-in-tree rescue, Johnny is using a black pen. But at the hospital after bringing tree-boy in to Rampart, the trusty green pen is in his shirt pocket.

Speaking of the tree rescue, I wondered how they were able to get the boy's BP since only his legs were visible. I guess there's a way to do it using legs. Something we don't see very often, at any rate. Also, when Roy was up in the tree and discussing matters with Johnny, he seemed to be shouting one minute, and speaking normally the next. Also, speaking of Roy, um, speaking..... I had to replay a couple scenes so I could enjoy his sexy-voice.

Another instance of creative time management with the tree rescue... when the sheriff took the mother to calm her down, the sky behind them definitely looked dusk-ish, I think I even saw evidence of artificial lights. But when they took the kid to the ambulance, it was bright afternoon.

Once again, Brackett and Early (and Morton) are the only doctors at Rampart. Today they hightailed it all the way to ICU to take care of a patient. Maybe one day Brackett will get the idea for ICU to have its *own* doctors.

I too liked the hotel fire scene. Roy was actually in charge until other engines arrived. Go, Roy!! Sometimes in these fire scenes, you can tell they loop the background audio, as you hear the same things over and over. Today it was noticeable with a man yelling "help!" and someone else saying "give me a hand." These guys knew how to get their money's worth out of both audio *and* video footage.

Okay, let's keep watch on how frequently we see Roy with a
book. He had one today in the opening scene, but he never
got to read it (he rarely does). The other day he had one as
well. Maybe it doesn't occur often enough for a drinking
game, but something to keep an eye out for.

Oh, and Dr. Early looked sharp in his street clothes. No
competing plaids and stripes for him!

* * *

> Generic location dispatch alert: "At the hotel" – 'cause
> L.A.County only has one.

When this happens, I usually assume the dispatcher just
alerts them to the fact that the building is a hotel, instead of,
say, a liquor store, or restaurant. The dispatcher has already
given them the address, so it's probably just a way to let
them know what kind of building they'll be dealing with—
how many possible people inside, available entry points,
what type of contents or floorplan the building has, etc.
Again, that's my interpretation.

> There is something sexy about the undershirts and the
> turnout pants with suspenders.

Um, in other news, the sky is blue and water is wet. HECK
YEAH, they look hot in their bunker pants, t-shirts, and
suspenders. Yowza, I love it!! I can't explain why, but it
sure does get my blood pumping. (And yet, I'm not sure
that seeing my local fire fighters like that would have the
same effect on me. Go figure!!)

* * *

The funny thing [about Johnny's kleptomaniacal act] is,
there was *no* hesitation on Randy's part at all. On entering
the office, he walked directly over to that spot at the desk,

and immediately put his hand on the mystery object. Almost as if he'd planned it beforehand. You have to wonder (well, *I* wonder, anyway) if they had to do more than one take of that scene, did he do the same thing each time? Or, again, was the object his to begin with, or something he'd seen earlier, and he just decided to get his hands on it? Unfortunately, it's another one of those mysteries we may never know.

* * *

I really hate the studio scenes. On Adam-12 too. You can always tell a back-lot "city street" because it always either curves away or ends in a "T" intersection with another street. In other words, they're not long and straight, stretching off into the distance. Also, they're usually very narrow streets, too.

"Elocution lessons".... yeah, good way to describe the other paramedic calls. As I said, it really does sound like they're simply reading from a script. Probably because the actor really is--gasp!--simply reading from a script. (Another personally quirky thing that I notice sometimes, and appreciate when done realistically: the radio calls from 51 to Rampart. Sometimes when J or R are in the ambulance, you can hear the siren in the background on the Rampart end. And we hear what Rampart hears--pauses, interruptions, ums, ers, "Hey Roy, what was that BP again?", etc. *Those* are realistic calls, unlike the sedate, monotone calls we hear from other squads. And as stupid as it sounds, I love hearing Roy and John's voice come in over the radio. Oops, did I just type that out loud???

~ ~ ~

Yes, this is the episode with Johnny's famous (or infamous) pickpocketing scene.

Glad I'm not the only one who noticed the "men in short shorts" at the college football practice. Also, I thought it had to be an awfully small college, as I've seen high-school football teams who have better fields and more people at practices. Where were the assistant coaches, the trainers, waterboys, and everyone else? College football might not have been as big a "business" then as it is now (witness the academic scandals we have in the news) but I'm pretty sure that's not how any decent-sized college football team (or field) looked. And LOL on the observation that the "22-year-old" quarterback was actually 40 years old. How funny!

At Rampart, when Brackett came up to Johnny and Roy in the cafeteria (patio?), they all just left their coffee cups on the table. (They've done it before.) Guess those firemen really are used to having other people clean up after them.

From there we go to Brackett's office and the afore-mentioned scene of Johnny pocketing the mystery object from Brackett's desk (which I believe was covered thoroughly elsewhere.)

Roy's sexy-voice is notable a number of times in this one.

For the call about the kid-in-the-tree, we hear that Patrol 69 is called out. Anyone know what "patrol" is? Not an engine, or a squad, or a truck, or even a brushfire unit.

Yeah, that tree rescue always leaves me scratching my head for a number of reasons... again, many of which were discussed on the other thread. For one thing (1), Roy tells Johnny, "BP has gone down, it's now 80 over 50." So what does Johnny tell Rampart? "The rate has increased, to 128." I'm no doctor, but I really don't think those two sentences are saying the same thing. Also (2), Brackett wanted he IV established as soon as parental consent was given, but when the consent was given, John and Roy just stood around holding the form until the kid was out of the tree. Lastly (3), was the chiseling really any faster than using chainsaws? If they only needed to cut that little bit that Roy did, why didn't they recognize that sooner and just use clippers (like the wire cutters or bolt cutters) as soon as the limbs were down, instead of standing around jawing about it?

As for the lady with the "styling orange bathrobe" (ha!), I thought she left again with the sheriff. I know someone was in the vehicle with him, and I assume the boy's mother went in the ambulance. I don't recall which lady had which name, but I agree that the red-haired woman who called it in was a great help to the boy's mother, and actually a great help all the way around. Hurray for her!

By the way, it was funny when Roy acknowledged Johnny's comment about the kid being "out of the woods." I'm not sure Johnny himself realized the irony of his words at the time.

Re the doctor who ended up dying... I noticed they used a chest-compression machine on him, so someone didn't have to do CPR constantly. We don't see that machine used very often. And yeah, another sign that Brackett, Early, and Morton are the *only* doctors at Rampart, since they have to rush from Emergency to ICU to deal with the poor guy. One of these days Rampart really should staff the ICU with its very own doctors.

Continuity error: when leaving Rampart after bringing in Tarzan (a.k.a. Tree-boy), Johnny was carrying the O2 canister. When we see a long shot (stock) of them walking out of the emergency entrance, Johnny's hands are empty. Cut to a close-up of the squad and Johnny stops to put the O2 back in its place.

Now the episode goes into Afterschool Special / PSA mode, about the safety issue of giving emergency vehicles right of way and pulling over, etc. And yeah, how ironic that Johnny pretty much described a dash-cam, about 30 years before they became common?

I too noticed yet another instance of someone named Charlie. Incidentally, the guy who played Officer Charlie appeared dozens of times on E!, often as a cop/deputy. Many times he didn't seem to have a name but in later episodes he was referred to as Scotty (the actor's name was Scott).

Add me to the list of those who like the hotel fire. Being first at the scene, Roy takes charge and tries to keep people from jumping or falling. And btw, what kind of mother drops her baby 2 or 3 stories without knowing someone is down below waiting for it??? That was horrible. Also, do people really wear those pink long-johns like that one guy had on? He looked like Angie DeMeo, but if it was him, he's *really* uncredited on this one. Also, it seemed to me like Roy and John were taking their time checking the 3rd floor. Just sort of sauntering from room to room like they had all the time in the world. I love the (hippie?) couple who were helping the old wino. And I also like seeing all the various firefighting equipment. About every four or five episodes, it seems the show gives the LACoFD the chance to pull out all the stops and show off its toys. Even if they have to do it in an awful, dinky movie set like the one in this episode.

About Nurse Gail... I like her too. I also liked Nurse Ellen who doesn't seem to be around much in season 2. Nurse Sally is pretty good, too. (I assume that student nurse Sharon graduated from the nursing program and was assigned elsewhere, far away from Dr. Brackett.)

* * *

118

To me [the item that Johnny pocketed] looks like a silver cylindrical thing. Sort of like a stamp dispenser. Similar in size and shape. In fact, that would fit, since the 'item' seems to match the rest of Dr. Brackett's desk set. That's my guess on what the item is: an old-fashioned stamp dispenser.

Or maybe it was some sort of fancy lighter, although it's not a very convenient size or shape to carry around. I just can't figure out what Johnny would want to pilfer.

Edit: I totally agree about the voice of the "other" paramedic on the tape. As we've noted before, every time we hear calls from other squads, they always sound so calm and relaxed, with no sense of urgency and no background sounds or noises... in fact, it sounds like someone reading from a script in a nice, quiet recording room.

* * *

Looking at pics of Brackett's office from earlier in season 2, I think the object that Johnny palmed is the round, cylindrical object often seen on Brackett's desk.

Again, can't imagine why he'd take it... maybe Randy just bet someone that he could steal something off the desk during a take and not get caught. ???? Incidentally, that object appears on Brackett's desk throughout the whole series, so obviously Randy didn't keep it.

2.14 School Days

The snake thing.... I fast-forwarded through that. Not only is it a cruel 'joke,' but it's a major waste of paramedics' time and attention.

Re the first call, of the man trapped under a fallen bookcase:

> One of my favorite little parts is in the first rescue where
> the housekeeper is next to Johnny and repeating the
> vitals when he's telling Rampart. Such a cute scene, and
> they both play off each other really well!

I totally agree... that was cute! By the way, Roy left his
helmet in that room when he left. Also, I know Gage left
with the patient, and I assumed the ambulance left right
away. Imagine my surprise when Billy got out of the
ambulance at Rampart... apparently they waited while he had
his chat with Roy in the man's library.

> Noticed a couple of our favorite stock shots, the white
> trestle bridge, plus they drove past the granary twice in
> about 30 seconds, ha-ha.

I know, right?? I guess Johnny just drove around the block
as they were talking.

In the ambulance rescue, I almost laughed when Roy said
"Cap, is there any way we can shut off that water?" I half-
expected Cap to say, "No, Roy, we thought we'd just sit
around and let it rain for a while." Incidentally I was
surprised that one of the three (count 'em, *three*) paramedics
didn't supervise the removal of the ambulance driver who
was pinned in behind the wheel.

Did anyone else think that maybe that chronic cough might
be harmful for someone who's supposed to work to keep
people healthy? I mean, germs do fly, after all.

And what about the old firetrucks at the junk yard?
Methinks we'll see them again in an upcoming season.

Roy might be married, but at Rampart I saw him checking out that nurse as they went to see the little boy in his hospital room.

Once again we see the senior paramedic take a supervisory role as he took the time to encourage a cautious trainee. And Johnny was good with Billy, too, they both were great coaches. At the junkyard, when Billy said the victim was in pain, Johnny asked "do you want to give him MS??" (Never mind the fact that they hadn't gotten permission from Rampart yet.) Anyway, I had the feeling that maybe he was testing Billy. And when Billy said "No, he's bleeding too badly and going into shock, I don't want to risk it," Johnny kind of smiled as if to say: "right answer; good boy!"

I do like this episode. I tend to like the rescues (the 'big' rescues, in the last 12 minutes) which involves the engine as well as the paramedics. I like when they all work together: everyone has a job to do, everyone has a role. Maybe that's why I like this show so much--the teamwork and organization.

~ ~ ~

I like this episode. Yep, I do, I like it. The only thing about it I don't care for is the "snake on the stomach" prank, I think it's silly and a waste of firefighter/paramedic's time. But other than that.....

One of the reasons I like this episode is that I like Billy Hanks. Other than Gil, he's the only trainee (or other ride-along person) who isn't a PITA. And he beats Gil easily in the likability department.

~ Billy was cited for valor as a firefighter. What does that entail? What do they have to do? Why wasn't there an episode about someone from 51 getting this honor??

~ This episode featured a couple of Roy's patented pep-talks, or 'senior paramedic moments of wisdom.' I like when he gets the chance to do that.

~ The absent-minded professor: his housekeeper was a hoot, especially when Johnny was on the biophone to Rampart and she was repeating all the vitals, etc. Finally Johnny held up the receiver as if she was going to give the number.

~ Lost equipment alert: Roy left his helmet in the guy's library.

~ The baseball player with the cracked skull: again with the injured athletes. Hard to tell how old this one looked since we never got a good look at him, but I'm willing to bet that actor/stunt-man was also about 40 years old. And I do have to shake my head at Dixie's conversation with the estranged wife... it sounds as if she was saying "yeah, you may have been going to leave him, but you need to stay with him now, 'cuz he'll need constant care, possibly for months if not years to come." That's kind of callous, if you ask me, and was wrong of Dixie to more or less try to guilt this woman into staying with her husband (and I'm kind of surprised she didn't say "hey, our fertility clinic can help you have kids, too!").

~ The kid with the science experiment: they never did learn what he'd been working with. Also, starting at this rescue and continuing with the others, anytime the paramedics were on the phone with Rampart we didn't hear Rampart's side of the conversation. Usually we (and anyone near the biophone) can hear the doctors' questions and instructions over the speaker, but in these rescues we didn't (Johnny relayed the instructions to Billy).

~ Billy's cough: yes, it was understandable and job-related, but I can't imagine it's advisable for someone to closely treat injuries and wounds if he's liable to start coughing uncontrollably.

~ In the aforementioned rubber snake episode in the park, as the guys all walked toward the victim, the dialogue we hear is apparently dubbed, including the chirping birds. We see Billy coughing, but hear nothing, and the other voices all have that 'recording studio' quality.

~ I like the junkyard rescue, and I like the guys giving Billy the chance to again take the lead. No ego on their part! I wonder if Tim Donnelly really knew how to drive cranes and other big equipment, or if "Chet's" experience with them was just the product of the writers' imagination.

~ Johnny sort of 'tested' Billy with that question about ordering MS. That was kind of cute. More mentoring by the experienced PMs--always nice to see.

2.15 The Professor

Not a stellar episode, imho, but it certainly has its moments. First of all, we learn that Roy's got a not-so-secret admirer. Of course, why he's so nice and polite and almost-but-not-really 'encouraging' to her is sort of a mystery, but, being Roy, it sort of fits his personality that he's not about to rudely tell her to buzz off.

Did we all recognize the house of Sir Erik and his wife? That was the same house--and same footage of the squad arriving there--that we saw in season 1's Cook's Tour, in which Johnny delivered his first baby. Let's drink a stock-shot toast to this house, which I'm sure we'll see again at some point.

Speaking of babies, I do like the baby-delivery scene in this episode. I liked the landlady being so concerned about the mother-to-be, and I liked the ingenuity that Roy and Johnny showed in creating their own incubator. Boy, I wish all childbirth was as easy as it was in this scene-- no sooner did Johnny get the gloves on (yay, gloves!) than the baby just magically appeared, no fuss, no pain, no blood, or anything.

Later, when they went to the dock to get on the boat, it's a good thing they secured the compartments of the squad. That way, when they get back to it later after the rescue, the contents will be safe while they wait for someone to 'jump' the engine because they have a dead battery. They left their headlights and flashing lights on when they left, and I don't think "automatic" lights that went out on their own were common in those days.

By the way, no sign or mention of Johnny being seasick this time, so apparently his earlier bout of it was strictly a (weak) plot device. And the plane victim... the audio we heard from him ("help, get me out") didn't match what we saw of him, the way his mouth moving, etc.

I had to laugh, when they got the call about the plane crash (I *think* it was that rescue), the dispatcher said it was "east of Lincoln, south of Jefferson." Quite a *presidential* rescue. They forgot the other directions: "west of Washington and north of Roosevelt."

Supposedly all these cases are 'based on real rescues.' If that's the case with the Sir Erik situation, I want to know what it was he was working on that was so darned important! I think it's safe to discuss it now, spoilers do not apply!

* * *

where Johnny was trying to get a date with the new nurse and Roy swooped in and got her attention off

Johnny. Johnny was right in saying Roy was being malicious and in that instance Roy certainly was.

Really? Did that really come off as deliberate and 'malicious' on Roy's part? I didn't get that at all. The nurse spotted Roy walking toward them and she turned to face him, literally turning her back on Johnny. Roy did *nothing* to purposely get her attention. I *was* surprised when she walked with him down the hall, but again, if she'd been interested in Gage, she would've been focused on him and not walked away (and it's not like Roy asked her out for coffee; he was only going out to the squad). Incidentally, that was the same nurse who'd been making googly-eyes at the pilot in the earlier scene. The nurse I *thought* we'd see more of was the one from the Sir Erik scenes at the beginning; she was very pretty.

I definitely agree that Roy should have been more forceful with the stalker girl. She knew he was married but called anyway, which was strange enough, and I certainly give Roy credit for openly mentioning his wife and kids to her, but he should have said "please, stop calling, you're disrupting the station and the hospital, and I can't have that."

Also agree that this particular writer didn't do John Gage any favors for the most part, which is too bad. And it is odd that he wrote episodes in which each partner got a crush from a rescue victim. I can't help but wonder, now, about the paramedic "Chuck," who Roy was partnered with when he met this girl, and why it is that the girl got stuck on Roy rather than Chuck. (Apparently Chuck has even less charisma than Roy, ha.) And of course you have to wonder if some part of Johnny thinks "If I was there, I bet she would have crushed on *me* and not Roy." I know, I'm seriously overthinking this, and that's too shallow even for Johnny (as written by this guy). But I don't think 'malicious' comes close to describing what Roy did: he walked down the hall, and was polite to someone who was literally standing in front of him. And, she walked down the hall with him. None of that was deliberate on Roy's part, because again, it was obvious that Johnny wasn't getting anywhere with the girl.

~ ~ ~

I noticed many of the same things-- a Chuck/Charlie connection.... Sharon being "heard (of) but not seen".... and the pilot of the fireboat also being named Charlie. Although in that last case, it's an honest occurrence, as I have the feeling that *he* was likely a real firefighter. (Not positive, though; imdb doesn't specify.)

For me, this episode starts off way better than it ends. The call to Sir Erik's house was interesting, Johnny was pretty quick to catch on that talking to the nobleman as if he were a scared toddler would help--not to mention sneaking up behind him to try to get the fireplace poker.

Roy made an interesting point. When he said he "didn't want to talk about it" (the girl thing), Chet called it evasion. Roy came back with: "Depends on where you stand. And I call it privacy." Very true--one person's evasion is another one's privacy. Then, when Johnny actually joins Roy and begins industriously polishing the squad (???) as Roy munches an apple, Roy knows his partner is just *dying* to find out what's going on, and he (Roy) gives this cute little eye-roll.

The aborted water rescue that turned into a downed plane... John and Roy sure do look good riding in that boat, I think. And I had to laugh at the obvious dubbing of the voice of the plane pilot, as what we hear is obviously not what the man in the cockpit was saying. Oh, and Roy left the emergency lights of the squad on as they went on the boat; hope that didn't run down the battery too much.

So Roy has a not-so-secret admirer. I have a feeling she must have been quite young, otherwise I can't imagine why she (if she was mature) would keep calling him even though she *knew* he was "married with children." And of course Johnny can't accept that a woman—*any* woman, of *any* age--would be interested in Roy, and he's not very nice about stating that, unfortunately. Even more unfortunately, what Johnny apologized for was *not* the fact that he implied his friend was uninteresting and as exciting as drywall, but just that he was tactless in expressing it. So what does Roy do? He tweaks Johnny's nose. A smile and a polite word, and Johnny's latest prey--er, I mean nurse--turns her back on him and walks off with Roy. T!t for tat... tie score. Anyway, even though it was never mentioned again (more's the pity), apparently all was forgiven on both sides. (By the way, wasn't that the same nurse who was making goo-goo eyes at the crashed pilot? Fickle thing, isn't she?? Not sure Johnny should even be interested in her.)

Chet has proven (both onscreen and off) to be good at talking to victims, keeping them calm, taking their minds off whatever is happening, etc. He was really cute with that girl who had her arm stuck the pool drain, too.

The final rescue was pretty boring, imho. So the scion of the wealthy Bentley family doesn't feel he can live up to what's expected of him. I don't know where he'd been being kept, but wherever it was he got away from, they sure had a fancy dress code. A lot of people can't be that well-dressed at their own funerals, much less while jumping off a building. And I agree, it made for an abrupt (and somewhat unsatisfying) end of the episode.

*   *   *

By the way, I meant to reference the baby scene in the tiny apartment. All I can say is.... Quickest. Delivery. Ever.

Yeah, the mother had been in pain or discomfort for a while, but as soon as the paramedics got there, they took her BP (not sure why; didn't seem very important at that exact moment), but no sooner had they put on their baby-delivery-gloves than--whammo!--instant baby. No fuss, no muss, either, their gloves stayed perfectly clean (never mind all the various types of goo that are involved in a *real* delivery). But I do like everything about the whole scene, from the really nice landlady (friend) to Johnny and Roy looking happy and relieved when the baby begins to breathe easier in the make-shift incubator. Even the ambulance attendant seemed glad about that.

2.16 Syndrome

Random thoughts:

~ Is this the first time we see Dixie in pants (rather than the old-fashioned nurse's dress)? It might be.

~ We see that Roy currently has a mirror on the inside of his locker door. (Although methinks that might be just a plot device.) In later years he has something else on the door, I think it was a poster from some arts festival or something.

~ Re the rescue of the boys from the tower... the call comes in at 8:10am, but when they leave the station it looks more like noon--sun high in the clear-blue sky. But the weather changes quickly in LA County, apparently, because when they get to the storage tanks, the sky is overcast and the streets look wet. Also in that scene, perhaps our cracker-jack audio listeners can find out something: once John and Roy come up with a plan to get the boys (and again, *they* have to be the ones to go...why, exactly??) they rush off to get belts and rope and while the main attention is on Cap and the old geezer, you can hear Johnny mutter something off-camera. I don't think it's scripted dialogue, but probably just Randy saying something that the audio picked up off his mic.

~ And by the way, why didn't they just climb up to the top, like Chet did, tie off the ropes, and rappel down to the boys from there? Wouldn't that have been a lot easier? And less dangerous??? I totally agree that R and J were great with the kids, telling them to be grateful to the old geezer, etc.

~ Lots of stock footage today. Looks like Happy Hour around here!

~ About Roy's tonsils... yeah, it was nice that Johnny was right... for a change! But really, who knew tonsils could grow back?? And since we've all been drinking from the stock shots, it's time to have some giggles over some of the dialogue surrounding the tonsils. Like Dr. Early calling them "the biggest I've seen in years." And Johnny saying "lots of people grow new ones." I know a lot of people say "come on, grow a pair," but who knew it could really happen? (At least for tonsils.) *wink*

~ And the final scene at Olive View hospital... I thought it was funny with the Battalion Chief telling that guy "stick around, the police will want to talk to you." Um, yeah, that's a great incentive for an admitted arsonist to stick around, they *love* to talk to police. Thanks for the heads-up, there, Chief!!

~ The firefighters had been looking for the missing two people for over an hour in all that debris, and it looked like they really hadn't moved from where they started, where Chet got hurt. But suddenly Marco conveniently finds something *ten feet* away.

~ Personally I didn't care much for Robert Alda as Dixie's ex. She had her "ex" ex lying in the hospital bed, when her current "ex" walked in the room (Brackett). To me, that would be like comparing hamburger to steak. (Yikes, did I say that out loud?) Anyway, maybe that's why she rushed out so quickly.

~ ~ ~

Not sure why this episode is titled Syndrome.... I don't think there's any single theme running through. If there is and I'm just not seeing it, let me know.

So Roy has a sore throat. For one thing, I didn't realize gargling could be heard throughout an entire building, even through closed doors. For another thing, who knew tonsils could grow back? I mean, yeah, I guess it's not impossible (obviously), but who knew that, and how often do you hear of such a thing??

So Dixie's ex becomes a patient at Rampart. After a bunch of tests Brackett and Co. discover there's nothing really wrong with him... except maybe they should've done surgery to remove that dead skunk from his head. And what does that tell us about Dixie's age? This guy is supposedly 46 years old, and Dixie knew him "12 years ago." It sounded like she was in nursing school at that time, but we know she was supposedly a nurse in Korea, so that's not possible. Fast and loose with the facts and dates again, writers! (Also, if he's some big actor, why was it such a surprise for these two to run into each other? It's L freakin'-A for heaven's sake.)

I like the rescue of the kids on the water tower thingy. That had to be an interesting rescue IRL. The old codger was pretend-mean about it, but he was glad to help the boys out. And the boys were glad that John and Roy were firefighters and not cops. Even though the difference between the far-shots and the close-up scenes was quite obvious, it was good and I liked the interaction between the paramedics and the kids. I do wonder, though, if, in real life, the boys would have been allowed to simply walk away like that, without any consequences at all. Too lucky!! (In more ways than one...)

By the way, I know it was stock footage, but when the squad and engine left for that call, it was bright sun. When they pulled into the scene, it was overcast and in fact looked like it had rained. Then the scene cuts again as they get out of their vehicles and there's sun again.

The call that took them to the women's field hockey game-- er, melee--was kinda funny. A little out-of-the-ordinary, perhaps, but still a little fun. I'm sure paramedics get calls like that all the time. And people laugh (or used to) about girls who play field hockey. Also, did anyone else wince a little when the girls kept calling each other cows? Today, of course, 'cow' would be replaced by the b-word. (Guys call women dogs, women call each other cows.... maybe the theme of this one is... animals??)

Meanwhile, back at Rampart, Dr. Early is treating the world's oldest grad student. In my opinion, Joe's at his best when he's working one-on-one with patients, especially oddball patients like our friend Dick, or the boy with the bunny in his tuba, or the man who's been cursed.

I think this is the first (and only?) episode that references an earthquake. For a show set and filmed in southern California, that seems a bit odd, no? And it makes me kind of outraged on behalf of all Californians that an almost-complete hospital building (I assume it wasn't totally finished at the time) is sitting empty waiting for something to be done with it. I know it couldn't be helped, but you'd think that planners would make every effort to discover where fault lines are before building things like, oh, I don't know, public hospitals are built on them. Anyway, the guys are still at Rampart when they get the alarm on the handy-talkie about the incident at Olive View. Roy finally says what I'm always thinking during those calls that include a bunch of tones: "This sounds big." Every time I hear a bunch of companies being called out, I think, "This is a big one," and I wonder why nobody ever comments on it. Guess Roy heard me.

Similar to the abandoned building rescue we had a week or so ago, this response is at a supposedly empty building but of course--this is Emergency!, after all-- they're told at the last minute that there are X number of people stuck inside, who were in the building for nefarious and not-entirely-legal reasons. So of course our intrepid paramedics have to rush in, this time with help from the snorkel truck (and a ladder truck was there too). After rescuing two law-breakers, they learn the other two are in the basement, stuck behind a bunch of caved-in debris. Chet gets hurt in the attempt to clear a path and gets a free ride to Rampart for a broken shoulder. Later after a lot of work and discouragement (I thought they were under some sort of time constraint?) they're still working. Marco used what looked like a Kennedy probe, but he didn't have the headphones on, so I'm not sure that's what it was. Long story short, this is our show and the guys always find the victims alive and in relatively good shape, all's well that ends well, blah blah blah.

That only leaves one piece of unfinished business: Roy's tonsillectomy. Maybe Roy should have encouraged that admirer he had yesterday, as I bet *she* would be in the hospital visiting him, unlike his absentee wife and kids. Instead poor DeSoto is stuck in the room right down the hall from the base station (?) with Chet. No idea why *Chet's* still in the hospital four or five or more days later, but this is TV so what can you do. Anyway, even though Johnny makes a special trip to Rampart to see his buddies, he doesn't do anything more than drop off Roy's ice cream and beat a hasty retreat. Speaking of headphones, Roy could probably use a pair right about then.

Odds and ends:

~ First scene: Johnny had a name-badge on his uniform shirt and also one on his blue jacket when he slipped it on before getting into the squad. First season, I don't think the jackets had name tags.

~ Is this the first time we see Dixie wearing a pantsuit uniform? I don't recall seeing her in one prior to this. (I think I noticed the same thing the last time this episode aired.)

~ Brackett had Raymond Boyd put in Observation 2. Really? More rooms?? Observation rooms aren't the same as treatment rooms?? Makes me wonder just how big that Emergency Department *is*, anyway. Sounds like Dr. Who's Tardis: a lot bigger inside than it looks from the outside.

~ Boot liked Johnny in this episode. But then he was only in one scene, so maybe he can only tolerate John Gage in small doses.

~ After hearing the tones for the final call, we see the squad speeding down the road as dispatcher Sam gives details. Johnny comments that Olive View was damaged in the earthquake, and then we hear Roy responds, "Squad 51 responding from Rampart Emergency." Obviously that would have been the case if they were still at Rampart and Roy had the HT, but once they were in the squad, Johnny's the one who would acknowledge the call. I thought that was interesting/odd.

2.17 Honest

A very interesting episode, for a number of reasons, so let's dive right in.

~ First off, did we all see the editing "oops" in the very beginning? The tones sound, we see the "real" FFs from station 127 running to the engine, and, lo and behold, Johnny is driving with Roy riding shotgun. But apparently they had a Chinese fire drill on the way to the call, because when they arrive, Roy is behind the wheel, and John in passenger seat.

~ Mrs. Epps, the mother of the boy who can't breathe (frog dissection) is the same woman we've seen before. Obviously she didn't learn her earlier lesson about tolerating child abuse, because now, partly due to her own behavior, her son is dead.

~ Since when do the guys have to go to the 3rd floor to get their supplies? Usually Dixie has everything they need right there at the base station (it all looked like their 'normal' stuff, too).

~ One of the nurses in the treatment room (maybe with the Epps boy?) didn't have *any* band (or stripe, or whatever it's called) on her nursing cap. I guess some nursing schools gave out 'blank' (i.e., unadorned) caps??

~ Aaron Sorkin must have been watching this episode and the lesson stuck with him. He even co-opted one of the lines. Chet says of Johnny: "you couldn't accept total honesty." In other words, "you can't handle the truth!"

~ After the pool rescue where Johnny was in the water with the victim, when he gets to Rampart with the patient, his clothes are no longer wet. Drip-dry material?? (I like that rescue, btw, not sure why. But I like the realism, with Brackett calling "Rescue 51, this is Rampart, come in," etc. Just a little detail that makes it seem that much more realistic.)

~ Funny, at the last scene at Rampart, Johnny finishes his cup of coffee (and leaves it on the desk for Dixie to clean up; thanks, Gage!!), and then as soon as they get back to the station, what does he do? He pours another cup!! What would these characters do without coffee pots and cups to use as props??

~ At the house fire, I love how John opened the locked/stuck bedroom door: by banging into it backwards with his air tank. Whatever works!! Also, I have to wonder, what did he think he could have (or should have) done differently there? If gramps had told him he was blind, I don't see that it could have made much difference. There's no way Johnny could have gotten both baby and grandpa out on his own, and the baby was the first priority. At the very most, John could have told Cap immediately after falling off the stairway. And besides, being blind isn't what stopped the old man-- blind people can navigate their own homes very well without assistance. It was the *smoke* that hindered him, not the blindness. That part of this episode always stumps me, as it just doesn't make sense that *anyone* (least of all John himself) should think that he "could have" or "should have" done anything differently.

And the question of honesty was good because it's an issue that's been brought up before on this show. The paramedics usually say "we don't know what's wrong with him," or "it's *possible* it could be his heart," etc., but they also sometimes say "your son's going to be fine," when in truth they're not really sure at that point. But they do know that keeping the victim (and family members) calm at the scene is usually much more important than worrying about telling the absolute truth.

* * *

BTW, since the previous episode was about Roy's charisma (or lack thereof), did anyone notice the way, when they arrived at Rampart, the house-fire woman made a point to grab Roy's arm, literally, and say thank you? Yeah, maybe she just thinks he's a hero for bringing ol' grand-dad out of the disintegrating house, but Johnny saved her only child, and we didn't see her grab *his* arm.

Also ****caution, shallow alert!! extreme shallowness ahead****I know we've discussed how, um, 'appealing' the guys look in their bunker gear, and when they're all sooty and mussed up, etc. Another look that I love is when they have full stuff on, including air tank, mask hanging (or clipped?) to the front of their coats, and.... their helmet tossed back, hanging around the neck by the strap. (!! *sigh*) I love seeing both the guys do this, but I'm thinking about it now because Roy did it in this episode when he brought grandpa out of the house. To borrow a line from Opie Taylor: "boy, I like that just fine."

~ ~ ~

The theme for this episode is honesty. Is it really the best policy? Is there such a thing as being *too* honest? The question arises at the first call of the episode, at which a husband lighting his cigar near a gas stove accidentally sets off an explosion. Although to be *honest* (heh), I don't think Johnny can correctly extrapolate that the wife's "little white lie" *caused* the explosion. Even if she'd been up front with hubby about hating cigars, that doesn't mean he would have given them up or wouldn't have lit one near the stove anyway.

But, however it happened, Johnny's on a truth-telling kick. And you know it's bad when he holds Dr. Morton up as an example of how the truth is always the best way to go; as Roy says (with apologies to Keats, I'm sure), "If you're holding up Morton as an example of the beauty of truth, you're nuts." Speaking of paraphrasing famous lines, Chet managed to do it twice to Johnny, first saying he "couldn't accept total honesty." And later "you wouldn't want the truth." Sound familiar? Put similar words in Jack Nicholson's mouth and you have the famous "You can't handle the truth!"

Not sure when this episode was filmed as compared to some other recent eps, but I noticed Dixie was back to wearing the standard nurse's dress. In Syndrome, which we saw last week, she was in the pantsuit, but now it's back to the dress. I wonder if the episodes were aired out of order. Or maybe Dixie simply varied her wardrobe? Speaking of wardrobes, the guys are back to wearing their jackets all the time, too.

I like the swimming pool rescue, although I felt really bad for the victim, who tried to do a backflip into the pool from the roof. From what was said, it sounded like the girl he was trying to impress wasn't even there watching, so not sure what he hoped to prove even if he'd been successful and hadn't gotten hurt. Anyway, this was one of those serious, tense rescues. I got a little miffed with Brackett when he was impatient about them not responding on the biophone. Sure, doc, like you're always right there at the ready the second Squad 51 calls in. Anyway, he knew Dixie authorized an esophageal airway, and yet he wonders why they're not responding to him five seconds later.

The fire with good old blind grand-dad... that house looked familiar to me. Reminded me of the house at which there's a fire/explosion and the one guy is dead and a woman is burned badly (I think it's Details). Anyway, at this fire, I agree that leaving "grand-dad" behind isn't Johnny's fault, although I don't think the woman would ever trust him again. But it's also true that Johnny ran into the house without any concrete info about the boy he was supposed to rescue. He told Chet to keep his eyes open for "a kid" in the house, but the "kid" was only a year or two old and wouldn't have been wandering around on his own. But Johnny didn't know that because he didn't ask. And it's not only the grand-dad who "lied" by not mentioning he was blind, but the woman did the same-- you'd think blindness would be the kind of thing you'd want the fireman to know as he rushes into a building to save someone. AmIright??

Also, when Roy was in the house and Johnny was outside stewing in remorse and self-imposed guilt, Cap said Roy would be OK and Johnny said something about him "walking around in a canvas bag." Anyone have an idea what that meant? Maybe the smoke is so thick it's like being inside a canvas bag? No clue.

Random notes:

~ Actress Anne Whitfield had lousy luck. In one episode her son was being beat up by her husband, and in this episode her son died, in part due to her own actions. Maybe her characters will have better luck next time.

~ This ep features two appearances of the Bird respirator.

~ Did we ever hear what the deal was with the guy who was turning 50 (??) and thought he was having a heart attack??

~ Mr. No-Charisma Roy displayed charisma again in this one... first he was being sweet and charming to the woman who brought in the car-crash kid, and then the woman Rochelle, who's grand-dad he rescued, stopped him and touched him and said a heart-felt thank you. I bet he could totally have gotten her number if he'd asked. (Sorry, Gage!)

~ The guys have the HT while they're in Rampart, but they also call in as Available once they get into the squad. So what is their status when they're at the hospital? Do they call in as 10-8 to Rampart when they arrive with their victim? ... When they drive from the station to Rampart for the ubiquitous supplies, they say "Squad 51, 10-8 to Rampart Emergency." That tells the dispatcher that they're not in quarters, but they're in-service (or on call, so to speak). So I'm wondering if, when they bring in a victim via ambulance, whoever's driving the squad and holding the HT will call in as 10-8 when they get to Rampart, so LA knows that they're available on call. And yet they're not calling in as "available," even though they are, so it's a little confusing.

2.18 Séance

This ep opens with the guys at Station 51 sitting around watching the movie Frankenstein in the rec room. And boy, didn't they look comfy-cozy on those hard wooden chairs! Anyway, between that movie and the main topic of the episode (and the episode title), you'd think that maybe this was the E! version of a Halloween episode. But you'd be wrong, since this one aired in February. Go figure!! (And while we're at it, the fact that E! didn't have *any* holiday-themed eps in the entire six seasons...? Who knows!)

Anyway, they were watching the movie when the tones sounded. If I were Roy I'd have had some fun with the guys and blasted the siren before pulling out—ha, take that, Chet and Marco!

So they go to a séance and meet the Teals. Nice couple-- he's in sales, she's in the psych ward. Or should be. On their second call to their house, it was funny to see how Johnny looked at Roy when Roy said sure, they'd look around the house to make sure there were no ghosts lurking about; I think John thought his partner was as nuts as the woman. But Roy had a bad feeling since he first met Mrs. Teal, so anything they could do to avoid something bad happening, was OK. Besides, they were already there, so what was the harm.

Two funny things about that middle-of-the-night call-- first off, it came at about 12:45am, and everyone was sleeping. But even though the dispatcher put in the call for Squad 51 only, *everyone* pulled on their bunker gear. Obviously that's another stock shot for the drinking thread, right? Secondly, for some reason Johnny came around the front of the squad to open the door and get in; it looked for all the world as if he'd just come from Cap's office. No idea why it was filmed like that. Afterward I thought that maybe he'd done the radio acknowledgement (KMG-365), but not only did we not hear any acknowledgement, but it definitely did not look like he was coming from *around* the squad, but rather from that door next to the map (which we all know leads to Cap's office). Anyway, I thought that was strange.

Coming back from that run, it was odd to see the night view of the squad driving down the street, with the interior all lit up. Kind of unnatural, I thought.

We got to see Roy putting tape on his pant-leg in this one. (Yay, I love that!)

In the final rescue, of the car trapped under water (with one of our fave stuntmen inside), did anyone else think it odd that the LACoFD boat or the other boat (coast guard, maybe??) didn't have some sort of air tanks or scuba gear (or whatever) that Johnny and Roy could use?? They would have had an easier time getting the guy out if they could both be down there for more than 30 seconds at a time. And, I hate to nit-pick with them, but they left the Jaws down there. (oops!)

I think that rescue was one in which Randy said he was cold and tired and just not happy and I think that came across after it was Johnny's turn to work under the water. He used the Jaws and got the door open and came back up, saying "the door's open." Roy asked "does he know?" and Johnny says "I don't know." His tone definitely suggests exasperation and fatigue. (Does The Book say anything about it??) And I did find it confusing... first of all, why didn't Johnny sort of pull the guy out, at least part way to demonstrate that the door was open, and secondly, why didn't the guy *see* that the door was open and just take a last breath of air and leave?? Technically, that's two episodes in a row where Gage left a victim behind. Oops again!

Oh, last thought-- the dispatcher Sam is like Brackett and Dixie... apparently he works all shifts, all hours.

*   *   *

I didn't realize they used a stunt double for Randy in this scene. Since the underwater part was filmed in a tank, I wouldn't have thought it necessary (controlled conditions, etc.). But yeah, I do remember him mentioning the slight electrical current, and I wouldn't be too jazzed about that either. I just thought it was an awkward rescue from beginning to end (no air tanks? the Coast Guard not at least assisting in the rescue, leaving the Jaws at the bottom, etc.). I know this isn't a 'true-to-life' depiction, but still, when something doesn't make a lot of sense, it's hard to take too seriously.

And you gotta wonder at the "powers that be" planning a water rescue for December. It's not like they couldn't push that episode back and deal with other scripts first during the winter months... maybe a rescue set in a nice warm greenhouse? Some guy getting strangled by overeager kudzu, perhaps??

Now that I think of it, this show could conceivably have used a "Frankenstein" approach to episodes: film a number of various rescues with the squad only, and then, based on how much time those rescues take, plug them in between scenes at the hospital or the station. Sort of a "mix and match" kind of deal. The editor could say "we have eight minutes to fill in the middle of this one... shall I use a heart attack, or the guy who fell off the ladder? Nah, we need something light and cute, so we'll go with the kid stuck in a dryer vent." And there you have it: cafeteria-style episode creation. Garanimals for TV.

~ ~ ~

So this is the closest Emergency ever came to a 'holiday' episode. It would have been good for the week of Halloween, but I think it actually aired in February.

We begin with the guys at the station watching Frankenstein on TV. I'm not going to comment on that movie except to say it pretty much set the tone for the episode, which was (purposely) creepy. Adding to the creep factor is the paramedics' call to the Teal home, where Mrs. Teal passed out during a séance. And let's give a hand to the melodramatic Mrs. Butler, who would probably be a 90-pound waif if she really lost 3-5 pounds each session. (Hey, I'd become a 'medium' if I thought it would make me a 'small.') Anyway, at Rampart the doctors determine that Mrs. Teal has no health issues and insists on going home instead of staying overnight at Rampart--a decision which her husband would have cause to rue.

And rue it he does, as later on (during the night) he has to call the paramedics again to help calm his wife. Mr. Teal asks them to humor her and look around the house, since the missus would believe *them* sooner than she'd believe *him.* Johnny's about to say "sorry, that's not in our wheelhouse," but before he can form the words, Roy says "Sure, okay." (Much to Gage's surprise, causing the 2nd of his funny faces in dealing with this couple.) Later, Johnny reminds Roy that they've done all *they* can do, as paramedics, and they shouldn't get involved further. Roy agrees, but he has a bad vibe about the Teals and wants to try to avoid something bad happening, if he can.

By the way, the above call was in the middle of the night, and when the tones go off, we see stock footage of the whole station jumping out of bed and into bunker gear (the same footage we saw a week or so ago--Mike and his blue boxers!). You could tell Randy was waiting for the cue, as he was "sleeping" with his right hand clutching the edge of the blanket so he could throw it off quickly. Also, for some inexplicable reason, the very next clip shows Johnny leaving Cap's office and getting into the squad from there.

The warehouse rescue was pretty much just filler, in between the Teal scenes. But it was a nice example of the guys noticing something amiss (distended neck veins, indicative of pulsus paradoxus) and being extra sharp acting as the doctors' eyes and ears. Also, we got to see a little of what happened at the warehouse in the aftermath of the accident, which was a bit unusual.

Later, Mrs. Teal finally does it--she's gone around the bend without a lifeline and started a fire. Maybe repressed subliminal rage against her husband, perhaps? After all, he didn't even go to her sister's funeral. But she's finally getting the psychiatric help she obviously needs, and it only took her setting fire to her home and burning her husband's hands to do it. Roy was right: that was some bad juju in that house.

Last rescue is the Beetle in the Bay. Or, Johnny Gets Fed Up in the Water. This is another one of those rescues in which (to me, at least) things don't make a lot of sense. Why didn't the fireboat have any light-weight air tanks for the guys to use? Their 'office' is a *boat,* for god's sake! You'd think that underwater equipment would be standard on it. Also, what was Engine 110 doing there? I didn't see them do a darn thing.

Quick bits:

~ The first time they go to the Teal house, Roy double-parks the squad.

~ One of the ambulance attendants at the Teals' was the actor Scott Gourlay, who sometimes plays a deputy ("Scotty").

~ Speaking of the Teal house, we've seen that same house exterior (or its twin) in other episodes, one being Fuzz Lady. As for the inside of the house, the layout of the front door, stairs, and the doorway next to the front door looked quite a bit like Major Nelson's house on I Dream of Jeannie. I'm going off memory on that, but I'm pretty sure the floorplan was pretty much the same as in the Teal house.

~ Johnny checked out a student nurse. Not Sharon though, she must have graduated by now. And Johnny's getting a little too old for the student nurses, anyway. But he definitely checked her out. **woof!**

* * *

Yes, I too noticed that the episode closed along with the door to the treatment room. As you say, it was a good touch, and effective.   Also, perhaps fittingly, this is one of the few episodes that doesn't end on a light, funny note. So maybe that's why, again, fittingly, it ends at Rampart rather than the fire station.

> Maybe the Jackets proved to be too troublesome for the continuity, and that's why they virtually disappeared in the later seasons.

I agree, that's a pretty reasonable theory. I confess I didn't notice all the zipped/unzipped instances in this episode, but I'm honestly glad they eventually ditched wearing the jackets so often.   In fact, I'm still wondering about the filming order of these episodes, as I remember earlier in this 2nd season, the boys weren't wearing their jackets that much.   Although I guess if some episodes were filmed in winter, they might need/want them. But what about Dixie wearing the uniform pants rather than a dress?

Anyway, other than the great eye-candy opportunities of them wearing the jackets over nothing but t-shirts, I hope they ditch them again soon.

2.19 Boot

> Roy was looking oh so handsome when helping the girl in the convertible.

You ain't kiddin'!! *fans self* I think the girl thought so too, as she asked if he'd stay with her. Does Johnny get victims asking to stay with them?? Not sure if I can recall a time. (Maybe the dudes? Ha ha!)

Johnny taking Boot's temperature. Ewwww! And he shook the thermometer afterward, as if he didn't intend to wash, sanitize, and disinfect it. If not throw it out completely.

The guy taking the aspirin looked like he was getting a red paint transfusion.

See, I was going to say ketchup. But red paint works too.

Dr. Early's watch - yes, I think we've seen it before as well. BTW, has anyone ever noticed how often Bobby looks down at his hands when he's talking? Or rubs one hand with the other? I guess it's his 'thing,' what he does when he has lines to speak but no prop to hold. Also, speaking of his jewelry, he had two rings on today. I understand that he and Julie either didn't or wouldn't take off their wedding rings, so now and then the rings are visible. I've seen Bobby's, but haven't really noticed one on Julie. (But then I haven't really been looking.) Apparently the rings are very distinctive... there are pictures out there somewhere.

In the gas truck/convertible accident, did anyone else see Chet's little dance with the hose when they first got there? It's right after Cap says to wash down the spilled gas, and right before the commercial break, I think Chet had trouble stepping over the hose. Oh, and we did see a patient with some blood on her, although supposedly her 'big' injury was to her leg, so... go figure why her face was bloody.

Finally, who knew "Klinger" was only 24? He looks older than that! And we saw another nurse without a stripe on her cap (or maybe the same nurse). And why didn't the other firemen see that man who was lying in plain sight in the burning lab?? (or was he laying? I can't think at the moment.)

Salvage covers - just canvas sheets? Waterproof? Fire resistant? Anyone? Beuller??

shallow alert I got another glimpse of the guys with their helmets flung over their necks and the air tanks on. *sigh* And they were all nice and sooty afterward.

Lastly, did anyone notice how polite and concerned Vic Tayback was about the poor convertible girl? ... until he found out she was gonna be OK, and then he started yelling and talking crap about her??

~ ~ ~

I'm not *quite* as enthusiastic about this episode as you are, but I still like it. I did find it a little unrealistic that at least four grown men (maybe five, since Cap joined in later) would worry and obsess so much about a dog that doesn't really even belong to them, and all go *en masse* to look under beds and in broom closets for him. As a fellow pet owner I think it's common sense that a half-day of an animal's moping and not eating isn't anything to get too worked up over. If Boot was still listless on their next shift, *that* might be the time to worry. And I confess I skipped most of the Boot discussion at Rampart. Even though there weren't any rants or silly physical comedy, I think this is a perfect example of the writers taking an ordinary minor situation and turning it into an extra-ordinary major Big Deal.

> Dr. Morton asks all the right questions – "Has he had his shots? Has he been wormed?" – before he remembers who he is and recommends not getting involved.

Ha, too funny!

The Lady Who Cooked Too Much was an interesting segment. It makes two episodes in a row in which the guys are called multiple times to deal with the same person. In a future season there will be the guy who had to be rescued while biking, jogging, and building a wine cellar. Off the top of my head, these are the only three instances I can think of. Anyway, in both Séance and Boot, the first two calls involve only the paramedics, whereas the third one includes the engine, as there are fires in both instances. Incidentally, I never understood the mindset that if you're going to do something you've never done before--i.e., cook--you should automatically set your sights at the very top, something really complicated. Why not make a simple casserole, or spaghetti, or baked chicken? Sort of like Johnny attempting one of the fanciest recipes from that Chef's book. I guess the motto for these writers is "anything worth doing is worth *really* overdoing."

By the way, after the wannabe chef said she dialed the phone with a fork, I noticed the phone was still off the hook. Wouldn't it be making that awful beeping sound?? And I had to chuckle at the janitor/gardener/handyman guy they kept running into on the way to and from her apartment. And then to and from... and to and from.

Getting back to the Boot thing, I had to laugh again when the discussion in the hallway at Rampart was breaking up and Morton said "This is a hospital. A dog??" You're right, Mike, Rampart doctors shouldn't waste their time trying to diagnose a dog. You need to hold out for a *goat*

Yeah, it's kinda funny (not) how the oil tanker driver is so concerned about the young girl... until he finds out she's gonna be okay, at which time he begins to blame her for everything. And this was another instance of nobody answering the guy when he kept asking "is she gonna be okay? is she gonna be okay?" Usually R or J or even Cap will just spout the usual "they'll be fine," or even "we're doing everything we can," but this time nobody said that. Did it never occur to these guys that if they'd just go ahead and answer the Annoying Repetitive Bystander, that person will *quit asking??*

I didn't think the Rampart outbuilding explosion was that bad. It was cheesy in many ways, yes, but it was a chance to show the LACoFD in operation, even if it was a little too dark and spread out to see too much. Also: salvage covers. I'm always surprised when I see this scene, that apparently salvage covers are nothing more than tarps that protect things from water (and maybe fire?). Also, I thought the burning vehicle in front of K8 was kind of funny... it looked like it was from the early '50s, towed in from the junkyard just so it could be set on fire. (Which it probably was.)

When the squad first pulled in at this scene--and in the prime, on-camera parking spot, I might add--it sounds for all the world as if Johnny says "Hey, Brackett, you need us?" The closed-captioning indicates that he says "Doctor Brackett," but honestly that's not what it sounds like. Just an audial illusion, possibly, but still I thought it was funny.

Quick bits:

~ Not only did Johnny drive, but he did it more than once! And bad editing didn't ruin it, either. Yay!

~ Did anyone see Chet dance (or wrestle?) with the hose at the scene of the tanker accident?

~ Dixie was in her pantsuit again.* And... no jackets for the guys. Another yay.

~ About the Jamie Farr scene, I believe I heard it was originally supposed to be in Helpful, but was cut from that episode, for some reason. And apparently inserted into this one. *Dixie's wearing her dress in this Klinger scene, so obviously filmed at another time and for another episode.

~ Interesting that another scene got cut from this ep, about Johnny buying a dog-care book. I wonder if that's why they had time for the Jamie Farr scene? (Eh, maybe not.)

ETA: Poor Chet, studying for the engineer's exam again. He seems to have studied so hard and for so long (lots of episodes), and he didn't come close to getting a qualifying grade.

2.20 Rip Off

Or, the *other* episode in which John and Roy discover they could be in bad legal trouble. (Yeah, yeah, in the other one, it's just Roy who finds himself in the hot seat, when he was accused of hitting the old man with the squad and the detective sticks to them like glue.)

Anyhoo.... first rescue takes place a little after 12 noon... and there's a wild party going on in the apartment building?? This isn't the first time we've seen rescues at parties that take place during the middle of the day. Other than the occasional back-yard cook-out, how often do adults throw adult-type parties in the middle of the day? Also at this rescue, we see Johnny do the "initial chest-thump" before doing chest compressions. Apparently it was at one time standard practice to do that, but now it just looks weird. Oooh, also, we saw *both* Roy and Johnny do the double thumb-flip with the medications, one with epinephrine, and the other isoproterenol (complete with orange ID label).

As for the possible legal troubles they were facing, again the question arises of the union rep. Or, lack thereof, I guess. And when they visit the lawyer, I know we all did one of these: :-o at Johnny's pants. (And we thought *Brackett* got dressed in the dark.... Sheesh!)

The car crash with the pregnant woman: It was funny to see Stoker dabbing at the blood on the head wound. Not sure how much help that was, but it gave him something to do. And when they filmed that baby-delivery scene, ya gotta wonder what Kevin and Randy were *really* doing under that sheet. Maybe thumbing through an issue of Playboy? Dealing a hand of cards??

Later, at the hospital, it was ironic (and poor choice of words) when the new mother asked about her husband. Brackett was telling her he didn't know anything as the husband hadn't been brought in yet, but his response to her was "I'm sorry." Can you imagine?? You ask an ER doctor about your loved one who'd been in a car accident, and the doctor says "I'm sorry"??? I know what that implies, right?? Sheesh, and he talks about Morton's bedside manner. Also, the hospital segments brought us an instance of a "Dr. Jose Estrada" page.

I like the plane rescue, it was certainly different. Who knew that going up (or climbing down) to get help could be so dangerous? Except that when they were in the plane (again, why did it have to be the paramedics who went in?? Nothing could be done for the pilot in the plane, and there was other non-paramedic-y stuff that needed to happen in there). Anyway, when Roy went back to plug up whatever it was he was plugging up, it seemed like Johnny was shouting, but Roy was just talking. I remember something similar at another rescue, can't remember which one, but one person seemed to be shouting and the other one didn't.

*   *   *

Roy and John had only the woman's word for the fact that there was a passed-out man in that apartment, so they busted in the door. What if she'd been wrong and there was nobody in there? Or he was perfectly fine? The LACoFD would be responsible financially for the door, and the paramedics might even have been charged with B and E. (In real life you hear about SWAT teams busting into the wrong house, so I bet cops and firefighters have some sort of immunity from prosecution in those cases. I would hope, anyway.)

* * *

I like Johnny wanting to talk to Joanne when he gets the good news.

Yeah, that's a hoot! He was just so excited about being off the hook, he wanted to share the news. And the look Roy gave him when he said it... priceless!

I can imagine they really were sweating it.... they work 24 on, then at least 48 off (hours, that is), so that's at least a couple of days of having this hanging over them, it couldn't have been fun. I'm sure the relief was like a godsend. Hence, Johnny's excitement to talk about it, even if he has to 'borrow' Roy's wife to do it. (Although there was a station full of guys who were also very interested, I'm sure. And Rampart does have more than one phone. I imagine even Chet would have been glad to hear they weren't going to be charged.)

Were they under arrest in the beginning? I didn't think so, but they got read their rights. At least the chief was there. Love how the detective was telling them to basically prove that someone else did it. They needed to prove their innocence, not solve the case for the cops.

Yeah, I too wondered about them being read their rights (that would have freaked me out!!), but regardless of the union rep thing, at least it was nice that the Chief was there (he took leave from his job as Lieutenant at LAPD to be at station 51 with them). It was kind of nice to see him be there for his men. (Although Roy didn't get that courtesy when he was accused of running over the Lighter-Than-Air man.) As for the detectives, yeah, I wanted either Johnny or Roy to tell them "we don't have to prove who did it, that's *your* job." And really, who does carry that much money on him? He was only across the hall at a party... was he looking to score some coke while he was there? Maybe *that's* what the cops should be investigating.

> Dixie's peach lipstick gives me flashbacks of my mom's Avon samples. I still say that Kevin is wearing lipstick or gloss. It's distracting.

Yeah, I have to admit I've noticed Kevin's 'glossy' lips from time to time, I wish they wouldn't do that. But maybe he had chapped lips IRL, I think he's a 'mouth-breather,' so that sometimes happens. And Dixie with her peach Avon lipstick. I remember that from back in the day, the women wearing the nude or pale lip color (although I hate women today wearing bright red--ugh! looks awful, imho). I remember as a kid while watching our Friday night TV shows, seeing all those commercials for Yardley of London makeup and stuff. Also, that was back when women wore the light blue eye shadow, very pale. Anyone remember that? In fact, I swear I even remember seeing Victoria Barkley wear blue eyeshadow on The Big Valley. (You know it's bad when the women on the TV westerns are made up in the popular style of the time the show was made, rather than the time when it was set. Like Miss Kitty with her long false eyelashes. Who knew they were so readily available in the 1870s??)

~ ~ ~

This episode, along with Lighter-Than-Air Man, shows our favorite FF/PMs as they possibly face legal trouble. Like, *big* legal trouble. I'm sure it happens in real life from time to time (it was a plotline in an episode of Adam-12, too), and hopefully those real-life instances are just as erroneous as this episode was.

Anyway, the guys are accused of stealing a bunch of dough from a TV news guy. A 45-year-old TV personality who had a full head of grey hair... which never happens, by the way. I mean, it wasn't even handsomely silver hair, like Joe Early; it was just a dull greyish-white and kind of dry and frizzy. No TV guy worth his salt is going to look like that! Of course, this whole situation led to Johnny and Roy being grilled by police detectives about the incident. (Note: I'm not going to talk about the union rep/lawyer situation again, as that was thoroughly hashed out in previous threads.) But suffice it to say that the Battalion Chief was firmly on their side... right up until the point when he wouldn't be, if they got formally charged. BTW, I felt like there might have been something we missed, some scene that was cut or something, between the time when Cap tells them "Those detectives want to talk to you and the Chief is en route" and a second later when there's a very unusual scene segue and we see Roy, John, and the Chief talking between the squad and the engine. Anyway, it was very abrupt and they never jump scenes like that on this show.

Ultimately, after a lot of worry, some lost sleep, a visit to a lawyer, and Johnny apparently being so upset that he loses all common sense when it comes to his wardrobe, the guys are cleared when it's revealed that the nice little old lady who let them into the building swiped the dough when her neighbor passed out. We'll see what kind of a neighbor she is when she's in Sybil Brand Institute trading smokes for a comb.

Getting back to their real jobs now... I like most of the rescues in this episode. The TV personality guy was a good one, alleged theft notwithstanding. And the car accident was interesting too. Although I did get tired of hearing that woman continually yelling for her husband. For god's sake, woman, they've told you repeatedly that he's in good hands, and you keep yelling for him anyway. And get this: hubby's name was Mike. There are already two Mikes on this show, so the writers add another one? What, they forgot that 'Charlie' is their go-to guy's name?? (I bet Charlie wasn't considered sophisticated enough for a doctor. Instead it's for lowly firemen and mechanics.)

At Rampart, Brackett was visiting with the wife, who was glad to have her baby in an incubator (which, sadly, was not made of a dresser drawer and plastic raincoat). Anyway, she asked Brackett if he had any news of her husband, and what does he say? "I'm sorry." That is *not* what you want to hear a doctor say when you ask how a patient is. In this case, Brackett didn't mean the guy was dead, just that he hadn't heard anything. Oddly, she seemed to know what he meant, but believe me, it always hits me like a ton of bricks whenever I see this episode. (Also, Kel told her that accidents like this often cause premature labor, but she told Roy and Johnny that they were on their way to the hospital already when the accident happened.)

The final rescue was sort of interesting, although maybe a little anticlimactic. Not quite up to par with other "final" calls, imo. For one thing, not sure how Cap knew that was liquid oxygen rather than some other fluid all over the tarmac. Secondly, he never got on his HT to tell 127 about the liquid oxygen; you'd think that when the least little weight/pressure could cause an explosion, a little detail like that would be of some interest when you have a four-ton vehicle approaching the scene. Also, I didn't really get what the heck Roy was doing in the plane. First he used some sort of plug for something, but then he had to shut off something else. Whatever! Most likely he and Johnny were thinking they were going to be arrested by the end of the day anyway. But I did think it was funny, after Johnny got the pilot taken care of, that when he went back into the plane to see Roy, Johnny was shouting, and startled Roy. Roy was speaking normally, though. Not sure why Johnny was talking so loudly.

Notes:

~ Love to see the orange/red isoproterenol sticker on the IV bag. Roy attached it to the bag, but when the guy was at Rampart, he must not have needed the iso anymore, as there was no sticker on his IV bag.

~ Johnny was scrunching his face while the Jaws were being used to free the accident victim. Not sure how he thought that would help if glass came flying his way.

~ Our favorite ghost doctor Jose Estrada was paged in this one.

~ The blue jackets were back.

2.21 Audit

Okay, I have to laugh at the guys having a coat-hanger (for opening locked car doors) and the anti-snake broom in the squad. What other odds and ends do they keep in there? At the end I was wondering if they kept any type of towels or rags in there to keep the interior clean when they're covered in wet cement, or crude oil, or mud, or whatever. I suppose they could use those yellow blankets they keep for victims, but that would be a little much.

Yeah, I thought Hippie George was a hottie, too. Just give him a good shower and shampoo (not to mention decent clothes) and he'd "clean up real nice." He wouldn't even have to shave, I don't mind a nice beard.

And I too have noticed how all the pregnant women are always "Mrs." whatever, or in this case, they just assumed that George was her husband. Here it was, the early '70s, with "free love" and communes and hippies all around SoCal, and yet everyone they meet is married. Even the girl who was pregnant (whose father shot her hubby) had just gotten married, even though she said she didn't want to. And of course there was that case in a later season in which the bride fainted on her wedding day, they learned she'd fainted before recently, and *not one person* questioned whether she could be pregnant. Well, of course not, because she wasn't married yet, and that sort of thing just *does. not. happen.*

For the most part I don't care for this episode, or at least parts of it. For one thing, I don't like the Wellman/Wells segment. He's a slime-ball. Worse, he's supposedly only 38. If he was only 38, then I'm a Victoria's Secret model.

Also, the whole "baby locked in the car" thing makes my skin crawl. Someone made a comment about people who are "too stupid to parent." Well, I think that woman at the hair-dresser fit that category. I know it wasn't illegal then, but still, I would have liked Johnny and Roy to stick around until the cops came and pressed a complaint against her.

The scene of Dr. Early with that Wells guy, he was checking under the sheet asking where it hurt. I wonder if Bobby got a little friendly with the actor on some takes, maybe grabbing where he shouldn't grab? And in that final scene where Early and Brackett confronted him.... Wellman's actions and speech patterns, etc., reminded me kind of strongly of Rumpelstiltskin of Once Upon a Time. I don't suppose anyone else noticed such a thing. (Yeah, I know, it's probably just me. As usual!)

Few other odds and ends:

~ Roy owed Johnny "four bits." Other than one of our cheerleading chants, who even knows what that is anymore? Who knew back in 1973?? (About 50 cents, I believe.)

~ It was so cute when Roy was talking about meeting the IRS rep and he said "we talked, we shook hands," and as he did that, he grabbed Johnny's (outstretched) hand and shook it. Too funny!

~ The chick who 'rescued' Mr. Wellman had a groovy shag-type of haircut. Sort of reminded me of Jane Fonda.

~ Johnny talked with food in his mouth. Is there a drinking game for that??

~ Did anyone see Marco with his "'stache-in-progress"? He was caught mid-'stache. I thought it looked good, too.

~ ~ ~

The last episode of season 2.

I have to admit there are some parts of this episode I don't care for too much. (And yet, I found plenty of screen-caps worth taking; go figure!) For example, the Wells/Wellman thing is kind of depressing, especially in the scenes with Brackett. Wellman is unpleasant and oily and with Dr. Brackett he acts smug and very pleased with himself. He *talks* about how much he hurts but doesn't *act* like it. With Dr. Early he's not so bad and at least pretends to be in some pain. Anyway, he's just unlikable all the way around, so I don't care for him much. (The actor who played him is in a number of other E! episodes, too.)

I also don't like the baby in the car scene. It didn't look like it was too hot outside (the guys and some of the women bystanders were wearing jackets), so heat wouldn't have been much of an issue, and I just don't like to think of babies being stuck in cars anyway. And then the shrew of a mother... bleah!!

I do like the story with the hippie couple, though. Funny, the carefree, heck-with-the-real-world, free-love, do-your-own-thing hippies apparently care enough about society to actually get married. And wear a wedding ring, which we definitely saw. (That's right, kids, only married people have babies. If you're pregnant, obviously you're properly married.) Speaking of that married couple, hubby George was hot. Obviously he could use a haircut, but I liked the beard and I think he had nice facial features. (By the way, I looked up the actor, and he died earlier this year.)

As far as I know, most of this episode (until the construction accident) happened on the same day, and yet Dr. Brackett is wearing two different shirt/tie combinations: a shirt with blue stripes and red and blue tie when he dealt with Wellman, and a different shirt with a tan and brown tie when he was treating the pregnant woman. And yet, I think those were supposed to be the same day. I wonder why, maybe the two segments were originally supposed to be in different episodes?

I like the final rescue, of the man at the construction site. It's a good example of a non-fire emergency at which the whole team is needed to help out. In other words, not *just* the paramedics. I did find it ironic, however... of all times when Roy and Johnny *should* have been wearing their turnout coats! The victim, Milt, was played by James McEachin, who we've seen a couple other times on this show. He played Lt. Crockett in a couple of episodes and was also in the final episode as the friend of the blues/jazz guy. In this episode he had a beard, though, so I didn't recognize him right away (actually, his voice gave him away for me).

If this rescue was based on a real event, I wonder if a real paramedic was faced with the decision of whether to cut off a person's leg or arm. What a horrible situation to have to face! Yeah, I know, it's not as horrible as the person who's leg you're talking about severing, but still, to be responsible for something like that is a terrible burden. I'm glad Roy didn't have to make a decision about it.

Apparently the doctors at Rampart keep a "go-bag" ready for times when they have to go out into the field. Other times we've seen one of them go to a scene (I can think of two off the top of my head), they usually scramble around for supplies and don't pick up that handy-dandy little kit.

About the whole audit situation... it progresses pretty much as you'd expect, since Johnny is involved. I thought it was funny when Roy told Dixie, "it took me 20 minutes to get him calmed down!" Just like a parent talking about a kid. (There's a funny scene in The Big Bang Theory on this whole theme.) Also, when Roy was telling Johnny about his audit, he grabbed Johnny's hand and shook it to demonstrate what happened. I thought that was really cute/funny.

* * *

About Brackett offering advice on the possible amputation of the guy's leg.... For some reason I was thinking about it as I was driving to the grocery store yesterday.

Brackett always says the paramedics are the "eyes and ears" of the doctors at Rampart. But the paramedics can only do so much, which is why the doctors sometimes have to go into the field. But until the doctor gets there, the paramedic(s) have to be the one to use their best judgement. As Brackett told Roy in an earlier episode (paraphrasing here), "Ask yourself: is there anyone here, right now, who can do the job better than I can? If the answer is no, you better pick up the ball and run with it." Well, Dr. Early wasn't on site yet, so at that moment Roy was the "most qualified person available" and it was up to him to "pick up the ball and run with it"-- that is, to use his *best judgement,* one way or the other. Nobody offsite could make that decision for him. And once Brackett told him to use his judgement, whatever Roy did was *technically* under doctor's orders, thus shielding him from legal liability. (Although we all know that wouldn't stop any guilt or angst that Roy might feel, so it's just as well it wasn't necessary.)

Season Three

3.1 Frequency

Another good "issues" episode, in which our guys (Randy especially) get to actually, you know, *act*. With emotion and everything. I think this subject was only touched on in one other episode, one of those brushfire eps in which a fellow firefighter is seriously injured while fighting the fire. That ep is Roy's turn to shine.

Back to Frequency. It's also another "pretty Johnny" episode. I swear, that close-up of him when he's talking to Drew's wife... he looked like he was made out of porcelain.

The opening scene was cute, how they were working on the squad and Boot stole one of their screwdrivers. Then they get a call, and leave the station with the tool chest in the middle of the bay. Bet the engine guys loved that when they got back.

While en route to that call (involving Drew), we hear one of the other squads responding over the radio ("Squad 59, 10-4"). We usually *never* hear any of the other engines' or squads' responses to LA, but since it was important to the theme of the episode, we hear it today. (We also heard Cap Stanley in that first scene say "engine 51 out 20 minutes" or something along those lines.)

At the scene... I thought Drew looked like one of the Walton boys. I know he wasn't, but he looked like he was. And after Brackett gave the OK for an IV, what did Johnny think was going to change in the 20 seconds they couldn't talk to Rampart? I know it was an emotional thing, and if he didn't know the victim he probably wouldn't have been so freaked out about the lag-time, but still.

Once they got Drew to Rampart, Morton danced with the IV pole. Actually, I think it slapped him. Brackett mentioned that OR would be on standby and he'd have to operate, but that OR looked like it was in the same hallway as the ED. And since when does a surgeon wear a stethoscope while performing an operation??

I hate to say this, but... I think it's so funny to watch Dr. Early 'rush' down the corridor. He reminds me of those race-walkers who walk kind of funny. And the young boy who was drunk... I have to say, I thought that kid actor did a good job. I always wonder how they get younger actors (under 10) to do some of the things they do, and do it so well.

When we see the engine leave the station on that final call at the construction site, we see Cap hustle into the engine as usual, and the squad and engine roll out. But is that really Cap Stanley in the roll-out footage? Sort of looks like the guy in the shotgun seat has a mustache. It *could* be Stanley, and maybe I'm seeing a shadow, but I wasn't sure.

Anyway, on to the thing that kind of bothers me about this episode. On one hand, John says that Drew was a "really close friend," but on the other hand, the wife says "we haven't seen you in months." Well, I guess that sort of thing happens when friends can't see each other as much as they'd like. Then, after Johnny took the phone call from Pam and was telling Roy about it, I thought Roy was going to say something like "don't get too involved in her life right now," or words to that effect. It was possible for Johnny to go overboard with spending time with her, and that would not have been good for either of them, for a variety of reasons, so it would have been wise for Roy to say something like that. Also, it bothered me when Johnny said "I tried so hard to get his death out of my mind, and then she calls." Well, isn't that nice for you, that you could put Drew's death out of your head after a couple of days and go on with your life. Pam doesn't have that luxury: she has to live with it-- every minute of every day. Unfortunately, it's something we all do. When we go to the funeral of an acquaintance, or a co-worker's family member, we all feel badly for them, and sympathize... and then leave there and go on with our lives. It's human nature. But the family members don't have that luxury to shrug and go on to something else. It would have been nice to hear Johnny acknowledge that it's easy for him to get back to his 'normal' life after the funeral, when it's totally impossible for her. Ah well, it's only a TV show, it can't be expected to do everything. As it was, I think it was a good ep that brought up some good points for the general public to think about regarding police officers and firefighters.

Okay, rant over.

~ ~ ~

So season 3 starts off with a good, John-centric issues episode. Nothing goofy, thank heavens. I believe last time we discussed the possible filming date of this one, and whether it was originally filmed earlier with some season 2 eppies. And now that I'm thinking about it, in the season two finale, wasn't Marco sporting the beginnings of a mustache? And yet here he is, clean-shaven. Maybe it really was just a hiatus 'stache.

In any case, the first scene of this episode was really cute, with Roy and John working on the squad in tandem: Roy under the hood, and Johnny under the squad itself. They did a nice little 'tool ballet' as they reached for and replaced various tools, all without looking, I might add. And then Boot got involved and that was the end of the work. And it's a good thing they were at a stopping point or else the squad might not have started for them. But I did wonder what the engine guys thought when they returned to find the tools and creeper (roller) scattered all higgledy-piggledy around the apparatus bay.

The first call is what gave us the title of this episode, and all the emotion too. It gave Randy a good showcase for his talent... not to mention his chiseled good looks. His friend Drew was the victim, and Johnny was upset that a busy day at Rampart's base station might have made a difference in treating Drew (although rationally, I'm sure he knew otherwise, just as Roy suggested). But it was a sad scene when Johnny realized that his friend had died, and with a ragged, raspy voice, he said he'd tell Drew's wife. It was a good scene. (Although later he mentioned Pam and "the baby." That "baby" was at least three or four years old; but I guess old habits die hard.)

Due to the circumstances that occurred at the time of Drew's accident, Brackett held a paramedic meeting in his office to discuss prioritizing victims the next time multiple calls came in at the same time. It didn't totally mollify Johnny, but at least it reinforced that everyone was doing his best (ahem! note the "his") to give the best possible care to all patients, based on immediacy. As Brackett says, at the moment there is no better process available. Actually, I more or less assumed that's how things were done anyway, but I guess as the paramedic program grew it probably got more and more busy so that overlapping calls became a regular thing.

Switching gears to the gang-fight, I thought it was interesting that the paramedics were asked to help out. Guess they called in as unavailable? We meet the never-before-seen Stevens, who is helping Brackett and student nurse Sharon 2.0. Angie DeMeo plays either a doctor or an orderly, not sure which, as he stops and assesses one of the gangbangers who's brought in and sends him down to the morgue; later he assists in breaking up the brawl. (Fun fact: the gang member Brackett was treating, the one who was afraid of needles, went on to be the voice of Principal Moss on King of the Hill.)

After the brawl, when John and Roy were standing with Dixie, it was funny to see Johnny jump when the HT beeps at him.

Also funny, at the artist's workshop, when Johnny asks about buying a small sculpture, and Oona says "they're reasonable, you can make payments." Johnny's look says it all: "payments? If the price was reasonable, I wouldn't need to make payments!" Also love Roy's little speech about how he doesn't like modern art, or listen to rock-n-roll, smoke pot, he showers every day, etc. Ha, I wonder if there was more to that or if any part of it was unscripted, or if Kevin had trouble keeping a straight face, etc.

At the final rescue at the construction site, Roy's the one who inadvertently knocked down the "house of cards" on Cap and Chet on the stairway. And since the ladder truck was there, why didn't those two just go back down to the ground and up the ladder?? In any case, Johnny was determined not to lose another victim, and we heard and saw how busy Rampart was at the time of this call. A bike accident with a fatality and a head injury, and a pulmonary edema are other calls that Brackett (and then Early) are dealing with in addition to 51's case. It got a trifle hairy with three serious calls all at once, but we know how it ended. In the end, there were no additional fatalities of the three calls, so it was a good day.

I still have the same quibble here that I had the last time around, and that was when Johnny mentioned that he had just managed to get Drew's death out of his mind when Pam called him and brought it all back. I know what he means, and I'm not faulting his humanness, but I think Johnny should have acknowledged that while *he* may be able to "put it aside" and move on, Pam will never be able to do that. Not saying that his feelings are wrong or unimportant, but he should recognize that his grief isn't quite in the same ballpark as hers.

Quickly:

~ Did anyone notice that Brackett said he'd have to do a laparotomy on Drew? Just like the one on Ellen Rockstraw's illegitimate son.

~ Dixie said they had an OR ready for Drew, but it looked like they operated in the treatment room.

~ Love the little boy who ended up being drunk! Well, not loving that he was drunk, but I thought he did a great job, and Dr. Early was cute with him and his friend.

3.2 The Old Engine

I agree that it was nice to hear the guys appreciate the dedication and service of the old engine (and the firemen who rode on her... although that sounds dirty!). But we saw that junkyard (and that engine, as well as others) in another rescue.

It was nice seeing "Big Red" for the first time. And funny when John and Roy were riding on the tailboards--when we see their faces, they're standing close together. But when the shot is from far away (behind them), the two people on the back of the engine are standing farther apart.

> I also liked the way they handled the rescue with the girl
> on acid. Johnny got quite a workout on this one, running
> down the street, and then having to climb all of those
> stairs, ha!

Yeah, on Adam-12 it's sort of a running joke (heh, 'running'— get it??) that Reed does all the chasing, and in this ep, Gage got his turn. However, it was *Roy* who ran up all those stairs, which was only fair so that Johnny could get to rest as he rode up the elevator.

Two fun facts: that same building was also used in a scene of an Adam-12 episode. Also, across the street from this building we can see a place called Funky Flipper Arcade. Is that a classic '70s-era California name, or what??

By the way, I guess that gunshot-wound guy at Rampart was nekkid under that little green sheet as he was being examined. And he gave us quite a good show as they were "scooting" him onto a gurney.

I too really liked the final fire and rescue. Love seeing all the teamwork and efficiency that these guys show. By this time (the 3rd season) it was probably a lot easier to get LACoFD permission to 'borrow' other engines to film these things, as it was nothing but good PR (not to mention good training). And I loved when Roy and Johnny came out of the building all soaking wet and sooty and with full gear on. *fans self* I love to watch them 'shrug' out of their air-packs, or 'shrug' them on. I know I probably say that a lot, so apologies if my fan-girl fawning bores anyone. If I got money every time I gushed about them in full gear (or bunker pants), I'd be able to buy my own antique engine.

P.S. I think I mentioned elsewhere that this is the season of Johnny's hair switching from side to middle part, so let's keep our eyes open. And speaking of hair... I thought Roy's was looking particularly fetching in this episode. I think that OD girl would have warmed up to him pretty quick if she'd been more with it.

~ ~ ~

This episode is about both an old engine and a new one. Let's start with the new one, since we see it in the very first scene. For one thing, I call bogus on Johnny seeing Big Red for the first time when he leaves the locker room after getting dressed for start of shift. How did he get to the station? He would have seen the Ward LaFrance when he drove in, or when he got out of his vehicle, or when he went into the locker room. That "unveiling" scene was nice, but not realistic in the least. Also, it was neat to see him and Roy riding the tailboard, which of course is no longer allowed. Did we all notice that when we see R and J's faces, they're standing somewhat close together, but when we see the long shot of "them" on the tailboard, from behind, the two men are standing much farther apart.

The first call is to the junkyard for a small fire, which the guys handle easily. Chet/Marco's hose has a wide showery stream, whereas John/Roy's hose is much more of a jet spray. Then they used their pen-knives to tear open the upholstered seats. That's when Johnny says, "Hey, Roy...." and Roy gives him The Look. It's not the death-glare, I don't think we've seen that yet, but this is the "I know what you're going to say, so don't even say it" look. Oops, too late. Johnny said it and Roy was probably already thinking it himself. And then, bing-bang-boom, they own a 40-year-old firetruck. (Although Roy mentioned something about "the guy who sold it to us said...." But the guy who sold it to them was an auto-scrap dealer; how would he know the vehicle's history??)

The next scene takes place a few days later on their next shift as everyone's sitting in their lockers getting dressed. Right after Cap tells them their old engine has been delivered, the tones go off and J and R have to run. They barely finished getting dressed and yet they already have their little tool holsters on. I guess they keep them attached to their belts? If so, it must be tough getting them through all the loops.

The LSD girl's roommate is played by Laurette Spang, who we've seen before (and will see again, I believe). But I like this rescue because it was definitely different. After chasing

OD-girl, they drove past the Funky Flipper Arcade and then Roy flew up the building stairs while Johnny got to rest up in the elevator. (I bet Kevin had to slow down a little as he was pretty much catching up with the girl on the stairs.) On the roof, Roy was calm and solicitous of the girl, and kept her focused on him while Johnny got to her from behind. And skinned his elbow in the process, poor boy.

The paramedic call to the Win With Wilby guy was a good one, too. Things got off to a rough start as the victim had been down for almost an hour before they were summoned, and things weren't looking good for him. The guys did everything they could for him, including Roy noticing the man's breathing changed, and that wasn't good news. They managed to get him to the hospital alive, but ultimately he didn't make it. Wilby won't be "winning" anything, and that housekeeper has a lot to answer for. Also, this call came in at 17:21 (5:21pm) but when he's on the phone with Rampart, Johnny's watch says times varying from before 3:00 to 3:30. (I love finding those little details... I'm a nerd like that.)

Meanwhile Brackett and Dixie are dealing with the Indestructible Gunshot Victim. That guy almost flashed the camera when they were getting ready to scoot him onto a gurney. (That guy Wells/Wellman practically flashed us too a while back. If that hospital gown had moved just a half-inch further in both instances.....)

At the final rescue at the generic yet abandoned warehouse, it was interesting that Johnny and Roy went down the ladder from the roof to get their victim, but left the building by walking out, once the door had been sawed through with the K12. And yet, after they shrugged and jumped out of their air gear, they seemed to be dry instead of soaking wet as they should have been. Also, I noticed Cap was still giving orders to the other FFs, even though a battalion chief was on the scene. Thought that was weird.

Notes:

~ For the LSD rescue, the address was given as 2267 West Hill, but the number that was clearly visible on the building was 11044.

~ The old engine had the driver's seat on the right, rather than the left.

~ They had to shoot all new stock footage with the Ward LaFrance.

3.3 Alley Cat

This ep isn't too remarkable in most respects, but there are a few things of note. (One thing being, it features a cat having kittens. I love cats, and the whole internet agrees with me that kittens are too, too cute.)

~ The airplane crash. It was good to see Roy and John being sensitive and considerate to the girl, and it's one of the handful of times they come upon a victim who's already gone by the time they get there. (Out of curiosity, what do they do in that case when someone is already dead? Have the sheriff's deputy call the coroner?) But the girl, Angie, bothered me. When she told Dixie the story of waking her dad and her dad making noises like a roaring lion or elephant... and then she gave a roar like he did. She just sounded like she was acting way too young for her age. Then she said "I'm not gonna see my daddy again, am I?" She was supposed to be at least about 9 years old... kids that age have a grasp of the concept of death, don't they? And then later she asked her mother about that "funny hat" she was wearing. WTF?? She was acting more like she was 4 or 5 rather than 9. At least, I thought so.

~ The boat rescue. I thought it was funny that the squad parked in the middle of the boat access ramp. I bet any boaters who arrived while they were out on the water didn't appreciate that, they wouldn't be able to get their boats out of the water, or newcomers couldn't get their boats *into* the water. ... During the rescue itself, I noticed a glare or something in the scenes of Roy working on the victim, with the Harbor Patrol boat in the background. The glare was on the bottom right of the screen. ... Johnny wasn't using his green pen. ... When the Harbor Patrol boat took the victim away, they left 2 firefighters on the pleasure boat. This is a great example of the kind of rescue I like, because it's complicated and awkward and it obviously wasn't (couldn't be) rehearsed to death because there were a lot of variables and moving parts. It's also a good example of Johnny "directing traffic" while getting the patient extricated and onto the HP boat. We hear Roy a little, but Johnny talks non-stop in cases like this.

*   *   *

We all know that Bob Cinader was all about the realism and the 'naturalness' of the scene, and that's one reason I like this particular [water] rescue (among many others). Rescues like this can't really be rehearsed. Instead, as we've heard in interviews, Cinader and the writers trusted Randy and Kevin (and the other actors) to make the scene look and feel real. They had basic ideas of what had to be conveyed, dialogue-wise, but the actors' hands (or tongues?) weren't tied to specific lines or words. They did what needed to be done and relayed the information that was necessary, in whatever words or ways felt appropriate to them at the moment.

I agree also about the 'helpful citizens' you mention. That too is one of the good things about these scenes. If Roy needs a bystander to hand him the drug-box, he'll ask the person to do it, even though it's probably not in the script. Or if Johnny asks someone to hold the IV bag... that onlooker will do it, even if the actor (or extra) didn't expect to be asked. I realize I'm probably repeating myself and overusing the word, but details like that do make the rescues feel very *natural*. And there's a lot to be said for that unrehearsed vibe that makes the show feel very real.

~ ~ ~

I like this episode, there's a little bit of everything: humor, drama, hope, and tragedy. Some of the humor and hope comes from Johnny's new bunkmate, the cat who's having kittens. Poor Boot is in the doghouse for letting the frisky feline in the station, but all's well that ends well for 51's mascot. After all the complaining, Johnny was looking forward to seeing the kittens again, only to learn that mom had moved them. Which is bogus, of course, because it would take more than one cowardly dog to cause a new-mom cat to move her five kittens. But I bet Marco was right, that she wouldn't have (couldn't have) moved them very far.

While we're being introduced to mom-to-be in the dorm, the clock on the wall clearly shows it to be 8:43am. Yet when the tones sound for the plane crash, the call is listed as "Time out, 8:57." So it took 14 minutes for Sam to finish his call-out??

I like the plane crash, and I like how respectful Roy is with the dead dad; he gently moved him forward against the steering wheel. (Johnny did the same thing with a car crash victim in another episode.) Makes me wonder though, what happens next. Does Cap have to stick around until the coroner arrives, or will the police handle that? Anyway, Roy was sweet with the girl Angie, and I had to smile when she said she was scared and he replied "there's nothing to be a-scared of." Too cute!! I'll repeat, though, what I said last time around, that when Angie was talking to Dixie and later with her mother, she acted more like she was four instead of eight or nine. I'm sorry, but that took me out of the story as I couldn't help but wonder why she was acting like such a baby.

When they brought the plane crash victims into Rampart, Johnny was eyeing nurses while he waited for Roy, and I didn't see either one carrying the HT, but later on, Roy had it with him.

The man in the junkyard was kind of an odd but entertaining call. How often does someone in that commercialized part of the county end up with a foot in a bear trap? I'm a little surprised they didn't wash off the guy's foot before wrapping it up, though. I liked the sign that said "Horny toads, 35 cents, you catch 'em." Too funny!

Then there's Virginia Gregg as the emotional actress and her ascot-wearing husband. Dr. Brackett was actually kind and sensitive to her, even without Dixie having to tell him.

At the school gas leak/choking call, have we seen the guys use that suction thing before? I know they use a plastic forceps grabber thing at the frat house at some point, but that suction-y thing looks like it would come in handy. And I was a little surprised they sent the kid to Rampart, mainly because nobody bothered to make note of his name, nobody from the school went with him or signed anything. I find it difficult to believe they just transport random, unidentified kids to the hospital with no documentation or permission or anything. Even back then, before the super-awareness of school security came to be.

I really like the final rescue in the water. Although when the squad arrived at the scene, for one thing there was another Ward LaFrance there (81s) parked off to the side. But Roy parked the squad right smack in the middle of the access ramp, so anyone who wants to put a boat in or take one out-- too bad, so sad.

About the actual rescue, what was Roy standing on, since the water only went up to his hips or so? I certainly don't think the water was that shallow. But it was a tense and busy scene, complicated by the water and difficult access to the victim. Roy stayed in the water with him while Johnny contacted Rampart and did the other stuff. Toward the end, after Roy used the K12 to free him, Johnny got the leg splint and said "here's the splint," but then he immediately handed it off to someone else and got the stokes instead. We didn't hear Roy say anything, but maybe if Kevin's mic-pack got wet (which it did), maybe it didn't work any longer and that's why we didn't clearly hear his part of the dialogue.

Bits and pieces:

~ This episode was written by a woman. It was the only thing she ever wrote.

~ Dixie asks a student nurse to give a patient's chart to Dr. Early, then five seconds later asks the girl to get Early to come to the base station. Make up your mind, woman!

~ Roy tells the guys that he used to date a girl whose cat had kittens, and how she dealt with it. But in another episode didn't he tell Johnny that he met Joanne in the 4th grade and didn't really ever date anyone else??

~ At the boat rescue, as Roy is helping get the victim into the Harbor Patrol boat, one of the onlookers finds one of his tools or gadgets and reaches over to slip it back into his holster. (The scene changes at that moment so I don't know how it ended up, darn the luck.)

* * *

Johnny's hair is getting long, he's about ready to switch his part. In fact, during that hectic, chaotic time of getting the victim out of the water and into the boat, his hair was all messed up and almost looking the way it will look later in the season, when he does have it parted in the middle. (I think it's pretty much unanimous that this is the Best Hair Season, for both guys. Roy's hair has been looking positively adorable too.)

The guy in the red swim trunks was Angelo DeMeo, our regular go-to stunt man, ambulance attendant, hospital orderly, and occasional crash victim. I suppose the official story would be that he and Roy were standing on what's left of the boat (or whatever they had to cut the guy out of), but in reality I'm sure it was just a platform for the scene to be staged on.

I watched that part again (getting victim out of the water) and I do hear Roy say a few things, but his voice isn't nearly as loud as it should be, as it normally is. I'm pretty convinced that his mic quit working at some point (because it got wet?) and that's why he doesn't seem to say anything.

Someone asked how Dixie knew the plane pilot "did something brave." Didn't we hear someone say earlier that he didn't want to bring the plane down in a populated area? Or am I imagining things again? Anyway, for an accident like that, I'm sure the sheriff's office would check in at Rampart about the victims and could have told her the story. (But that's just me speculating, because otherwise Dixie wouldn't have any way of knowing what the pilot did or why.)

3.4 An English Visitor

Okay, so about An English Visitor. First, during the first alarm, did everyone see Cap step from the rec room through some small doors, directly to the little radio alcove to give his response? That was odd, I thought; not sure we've ever seen those doors open before.

Also, it was funny during that call to the Wild West Show couple, to see Johnny waving the gun around. You'd think he'd know better than to do that. Also, I wonder why they even bothered calling in to Rampart for that? It was more of a legal/civil matter than a medical one.

Funny to hear the Brit say to Johnny (in relation to the nurse in Orthopedics), "As you Americans say, Have you made out yet?" Now, I'm pretty sure that even back in the early '70s, a question about whether someone has "made out" (in reference to a girl) would mean something very different from what he was asking. Of course, he was asking in the sense of a general "made out," like when you ask someone how they "made out" on a test at school, or at the batting cage or grocery store. For most people, I think it means something a *leeetle* bit different when referring to a member of the opposite sex.

About the pot-truck that crashed.... you'd think the, um, *aroma* would have been immediately identifiable to a bunch of healthy, normal guys in their 20s and 30s. I mean really, it's a pretty distinctive smell. (Or so I'm told.) Of course we can make all sorts of jokes about how they'd purposely drag their feet in cleaning up the accident so they could inhale as much as possible, or try to sneak a souvenir into the pocket of their turnout coat, or even the fact that one of them should've said "Suddenly I'm craving tacos" (or brownies, or something, y'know?). But it was interesting that when Roy joined Johnny and Channing where they were with the victim, he seemed totally unaffected by the fumes. Maybe he was used to it, perhaps? After all, we know he'd partaken of some of that there wacky weed when he was in the "Narcotics Pit of Despair" back in the late 60s. *wink*

177

Lastly, in the final rescue, I wasn't sure exactly what happened
that caused the stokes to fall, thereby causing Johnny to lunge
after it and almost become a victim himself. (Which is ironic
because when Channing was allowed to go up with them,
Johnny admonished him to be careful because "we don't want
to have to rescue you, too." Irony, thy name is Emergency!)

* * *

> Roy, our wild and crazy '60s junkie! In this case, I think
> he's so straight that pot does nothing to him at all. A
> stoned Johnny would be a lot calmer.

Yeah, straight-arrow Roy DeSoto is probably totally
unaffected by the 'funny smoke.' He's totally immune to the
allure of maryjane. And I totally agree about John--give him a
few 'special' brownies and he'd probably be a *LOT* easier to
deal with.

> Even when you know that our star isn't going to plunge to
> his death, it's still scary to watch a moment like that.

I also noticed that we never actually see "Johnny" in that
scene. We only see the action from below--a firefighter with
dark hair wearing a helmet, but not his face. Never once do
we see a shot from over Channing's shoulder, with a view of
Gage as he dangles below. So, keeping Randy's rule of thumb
in mind, maybe that wasn't him at all.

(And btw, why didn't Cap immediately order Chet to scramble
up that scoop-stairway thing? It would only have taken a
minute and he could have helped Channing bring Johnny up.)

~ ~ ~

I like the way this one opens: the squad backs in and Roy is
obviously smiling, if not trying not to laugh. Real or no? Of
course, it could possibly be explained by the "great rescue"
that Johnny wants to share with the rest of the station guys;

whatever it was, it must have been both great and fun. Anyway, that's when Dick Friend (real or no?) was at the station and had brought a, er, friend: Jason Channing, who's visiting from England. I must say, I think Johnny was somewhat less than welcoming to Channing, more interested in telling his story than being polite to the visitor. Regardless, the station is called out at that point, and Jason gets thrown into the action with both feet. Structure fire, person trapped in elevator, and injured by Molotov cocktail. Yep, a prime example of us "crazy Yanks."

At Rampart, I thought it was interesting that Dixie told Squad 14 that "a doctor is en route." Also, we get another example of the "sterile" other squads calling in, in this case, squad 24.

Also at Rampart we get a very OOC (out of character) Joe Early dressing down Nurse Snippy in a room full of people. Maybe the writers just wanted to mix things up and Early drew the short straw to be the "bad guy" for a change. Dixie also got into the act, but later on she and the nurse made their peace with each other. Another Rampart storyline was the "rock singer" who was brought in by some random paramedic… because big rock stars live in apartments, right??

Next up for the paramedics is the Wild West couple. What did they do, tour with Jesse James back in the day? Anyway, I don't know why they bothered calling Rampart on that one. Glad they called the cops, though… wouldn't be surprised if their first instinct was to arrest Johnny for the way he was waving that gun around. And Channing nailed it in his assessment of the old couple: "You're nuts!"

Can't believe we actually see Dixie moving the markers on the status board! I still think it's a great idea but can't possibly be practical

Had to chuckle about the vehicle accident with the pot truck. Still can't believe they didn't notice and recognize the, er, aroma sooner. As for the final rescue at the rock quarry... I realize that the point of that whole rescue is to show Johnny in jeopardy yet again (and Channing come to his rescue), but I agree with whoever said that I'd have liked to actually *seen* the rescue of the trapped man. I thought that looked kind of interesting. And I guess the reason it had to be Johnny who almost fell was because he and Channing had been "at daggers drawn" with each other. At least, Johnny felt that way a bit; I don't think Jason did. Bottom line: poor Roy is left waiting with an injured man, probably feeling as if he'd been deserted. And I have to ask—again!—why the rest of the FFs just stood around like goobers while Johnny was dangling there? That never makes sense to me when I see this episode.

3.5 Heavyweight

First off, I know John Gage (i.e., Randy Mantooth) was good-looking (and still is handsome), but I have to say, I do feel he wasn't exactly built like a typical stud, so while he wasn't really "soft" (he didn't have enough "meat" on him for that), he'd never be mistaken for a gym-rat, either. Just wanted to get that out of the way.

Now, on to the show....

First alarm goes off at 12:46am, and we get a gratuitous (albeit totally *welcome*) glimpse of the guys in their boxers as they pull on their bunker gear. Woohoo, great way to start off an episode!! Oddly enough, though, when we see them from a long-shot getting into the engine and squad, they're magically wearing their regular blue uniforms. Must be that E-magic!

So we have the girl about to give birth under a black cloud of bad luck as she supposedly is being punished for her 'sins.' Well, boo-friggin'-hoo! Suck it up, chick, and get on with your life. And naturally they were careful to mention that she and "Rab" (nice name, dude) were married, and we even saw her wedding ring a time or two to remind us that these are 'good kids' and, more importantly, this is a family show (and therefore babies are *only* born to married couples, of course). By the way, they were apparently all in a band in that building, so I wonder if there was some of that "peculiar smell" involved, the kind we heard about in the other episode when the English chap was visiting.

Anyway, was it just me or was there a sudden and strange heat spell around the time that Roy got to the hospital with Mrs. Doomed? Boy, did he look hot in his bunker pants and blue jacket. Johnny too, of course, but Roy coming around the corner kind of took me by surprise... not to mention kind of took my breath away. Add a little soot from the fire and man, we're talking about a whole different kind of smokin'.

Speaking of the hospital, what the heck was a 10-12 year-old kid doing fixing a TV at 1:00 in the morning?? Of course the mother was so drugged out she had no idea what was going on. But Dixie prescribed her universal cure (coffee) and all was right with the world. (Except in this case, coffee probably was the best thing for that chick.)

And more hospital drama with the young woman not wanting her baby. Not only was there a lot of Rampart in this episode, but we had to endure waaaay too much of that insipid muted 'soap opera' music during those scenes. Very annoying, not to mention overused, imho.

We got a glimpse of the boys leaving Rampart, with *Johnny* getting in the driver's seat. (Yay!) I was hoping for an in-squad scene next, to be sure they kept the continuity, but no such luck; next time we saw them they were walking into the rec room at the station.

I know the engine got called to the apartment fire in the first scene, but we didn't really see much of the guys while there-- no individual shots of any of them, I don't think. So basically, there was almost no engine 51 action in this episode. The squad got called out with some other engine (85) for the hang-glider, even though that engine didn't get paged at the same time as our guys. Maybe engine 85 called for the squad once they got there; that's kind of what it sounded like.

Speaking of Glider-man, he said his right leg was hurt. The way he was positioned in that tree, when Johnny asked him "Where do you hurt?" I half-expected the guy to say "Where do you think? My b*lls are being crushed to bits." It certainly was an awkward way to have the victim stuck in a tree. (True story: I paused the scene right after he tells Johnny that his leg is hurt, and the closed-captioning on the paused scene has Johnny asking "Which one?" Man stuck with a tree branch between his legs + Johnny asking "which one is hurt" = My kind of scene. ha ha.)

*   *   *

I'm glad I'm not the only one affected by the guys at the hospital, after the fire. Woo, if I had to pick a perfect way for John and Roy to look.... the way they looked there would be it. Can I have a photo please, preferably a life-sized cardboard cut-out, just as they looked in that scene? That sure would be, um, stimulating to have.

Oh, and I forgot to mention something in my original post-- I think Roy and Johnny's hotness, not to mention my giggling at the glider-man's "private" pain (or *privates* pain," as the case may be), those things distracted me so that I forgot to mention one big thing. That rescue of the shooting victim and knife victim... I love the actual medical parts of that rescue, with our fave paramedics doing their thing. But the whole kid-with-a-gun scene, and him walking past not just one, but *two* sheriff's deputies with a shotgun in his hand?? Sorry, but that's just too unbelievable and stupid for words. In fact, the way that whole that scene was handled, even from the beginning when they didn't know where the gunman was-- from a police/law-enforcement perspective it's just ridiculous. (Guess I've been watching too much Adam-12, where those kinds of situations are handled with a little more attention to accuracy.) Anyway, it was only a TV scene, and a show that focuses more on the medical rather than the legal, so I think that's why I subconsciously just put the whole scene out of my mind and forgot about it 'til just now. But again, I did like how the guys each had charge of a patient, that part of the scene was good.

~ ~ ~

This episode is pretty much only so-so. Some good rescues, but also a lot of ho-hum stuff going on. I hate to pick on Rampart and say that stories based there are boring, but, well... sometimes they are. And this is one of those times.

Anyway, this one opens in the middle of the night, and the station gets called to an apartment fire. (By the way, meant to mention in English Visitor that it was a nice touch to see Engine 51 *not* being the first on the scene for a change.) But here, they are the first on scene, and as usual Cap dispatches everyone on various assignments until the Battalion Chief arrives. There was quite a bit of stock footage used in this fire scene, but one detail I liked, and that seemed realistic to me, is that most FFs are wearing air tanks, and we see two such guys run into the building empty-handed; turns out they relieve two other guys who do not have masks on. Seemed kinda fitting that the first two rushed in to get started on fighting the fire, and they 'held the fort' while others got themselves fully equipped.

At this rescue we meet Mr. and Mrs. Rab Something-or-Other. (What, the writers finally realized they can't name another guy Charlie, so they go with.... Rab?? Those aren't the only two choices!) Anyway, she's 8 months pregnant and all is well until she suddenly goes into labor. I thought Roy was awfully sweet with her; at one point, as she had her hand on her baby-belly, he put his hand on top of hers. It was so cute! Meanwhile, Johnny's inside helping to protect stuff with salvage covers and takes a fall, injuring his shoulder. He insists he's fine, but Roy looks at him with concern just before he gets into the ambulance with Mrs. Mom-to-Be.

At Rampart Roy insists that Johnny get his shoulder looked at and this begins the underlying theme of the episode. While both our boys look H.O.T.T in their bunker pants and blue jackets (and just enough soot on their faces to make them totally adorable, Morton gives John the once-over for his shoulder. Nothing too serious, although it sounds like he needs to take it easy for a day or so. The big shock comes when Morton calls Gage "soft." Yeah, you can imagine how well that goes over with Firebrand Johnny. From here, this storyline sort of parallels the one we'll see later on, when (again instigated by Dr. Morton), someone goes overboard with diet and nutrition.

Lots of drama at Rampart with Mrs. Rab and her baby and she believes she and her marriage are doomed, blah blah blah. Also, a brief story about a kid who got electric shock while fixing a TV—and his probably stoned mother. They were brought in by some random, nameless paramedic we'll probably never see again. (Second ep in a row that's happened.)

Getting back to our paramedics, they take a call that leads to a neighborhood spat that leaves one man shot and another one stabbed. Good catch on recognizing the daughter, Angie, as being the same actress who appeared in an earlier episode as a hooker who brought her 'client' to Rampart even though she didn't know what was wrong with him (he didn't speak English). But this whole call about the feuding neighbors is so ridiculous. For one thing, as soon as Johnny calls Rampart from the landline of victim #2's house, Brackett asks, "Have you started an IV yet?" Um, NO, because *you* have to tell them to start IVs, and you usually don't do that until *after* you hear the vitals, which hasn't happened yet. Duh! And then, the really, really crazy part is... the generically-named Tommy walks out of his house—which is supposed to be being watched by the cops—he walks out and walks past not just one, but *two* officers—carrying a rifle! The cops weren't even facing the house, but they see a kid walk past them with a loaded weapon and they just stand there. Anyway, that part really burns my biscuits, but other than that, I like this rescue. (Sort of reminds me of the one with the former soldier who has PTSD.)

So the final rescue is a hang-glider who ended up in an awkward position in a tree (hope he doesn't want kids). Had to laugh when Johnny arrives next to him in the tree and asks "Where do you hurt?" "Well, I've got a big, honkin' tree limb between my legs; where do you *think* I hurt?" Anyway, it's kind of an interesting, if low-key, rescue. Instead of them trying to lower the man out of the tree, it's pretty clever of them to lower the whole tree branch.

This 'n' That:

~ Couldn't tell about Roy, but in the first rescue (apartment fire in the middle of the night), Johnny's wearing his blue uniform pants under his bunkers. Wonder why?

~ Speaking of middle of the night, yet again we see that Dixie, Early, et al, work around the clock. (Incidentally, when Sam made the call-out for the apartment fire, he never did give a "time out."

~ Chet and Marco were at the table with some impressive-looking books. Studying for the engineer's exam, perhaps??

~ Rampart's phone number is 555-4667. Interesting that even in the mid-'70s TV shows were already using the 555 numbers.

3.6 Snakebite

Yeah, this one is fan-girl Christmas for the Gage Girls. It's the middle leg of the JIJ Trifecta: Virus, Snake Bite, and The Nuisance.

So, from the beginning... I totally agree about the "nice view" of a long-legged man in jeans. Yum, yum, very nice!! Now, not to be cynical, but is there really a point to putting out flares in the middle of the day? I always thought of flares as being helpful at night or in poor visibility. Also, was there a reason that Chet couldn't just take Johnny's Rover to get help? Or does that fall into the "duh, too obvious, dramatic license" category??

I do like the scene of "serious, no-nonsense Johnny" at that doctor's office. "Is there a switchboard operator?" "I operate the switchboard." "Then go operate the switchboard and get me an outside line." As we all lament here, we don't get to see Serious Johnny often enough. Both guys had their moments of Impassioned speeches, all directed at the nurse. And Dr. Frick was good too. As you say, I could have done without the Rollie Fingers curlie-cue mustache, but he was the kind of character I'd have liked to have seen more of. However, I did wonder where Frick's cousin was.... you know: Frack.

As for the "primary" sequence of events.... did we all notice the Amazing Changing Dozer Driver Helmet? It has a visor!

Now it doesn't have a visor! Wait, there's the visor again! It's magic!!!

When the copter was approaching the hospital with the three victims, you could see the chopper landing pad (the big red cross), but there was no ambulance waiting there. Maybe they had to walk the rest of the way??

I've noticed other times that the guys turn the HT around to be sure they're talking in it the right way, I know I've seen Johnny do it before. Too bad Cap didn't get the memo on it when he spoke into the engine's radio the wrong way en route to Rampart.

Speaking of the HT... when Johnny got bitten, he dropped the HT, and it slid across the top of the car to the opposite side. But a second later, he has the HT again. Maybe it's like Thor and his Hammer... it always magically returns to his hand.

I still don't understand why Roy (and maybe one of the doctors) couldn't have taken the allergy test thing and met the engine along the way, so that at least by the time they got to Rampart, they wouldn't have had to wait as long to administer the antivenin. It seems like a perfectly sensible plan to me.

* * *

All the times we see the guys leave expensive, specialized equipment to be lost forever... and Johnny has to go running down the hill for a $40 walkie-talkie.

(Disclaimer: I don't know how much they really cost, especially back then, but they certainly weren't as expensive as other stuff we've seen them leave behind.)

Looked like Chet was using some sort of gadget (shaped like a fat pen) to draw out the venom, is that what you meant? I mean, he wasn't actually trying to physically suck it out himself, of course. Not sure, but J and R might have used the same thing on the woman who was bitten by a snake at the gold course in the first season.

~ ~ ~

Okay, so it's the middle leg of the Johnny in Jeopardy trio. We all know that Gage-girls love it, and admire his "heroics" toward the end, but I'll get to that shortly.

For me, this episode begins better than it ends… although there is some symbolic symmetry going on at the two points. In any case, the ep starts with John, Roy, and Chet returning from a (futile) fishing trip in the middle of nowhere. Must have been Nevada or Arizona, as they're definitely out of state. They come upon an accident scene, and I have to say, this was the strangest accident I've ever seen. Two vehicles in the middle of nowhere on a straight road… and they just happen to run into each other. Johnny gets out and runs to the pickup truck, but the driver is dead. And note that the truck's windshield is gone—it's lying practically in one piece on the truck's hood. Maybe this is one of those strange spots on the earth where the laws of physics don't apply? The second car has a mother in the front seat and a boy—at least 8 or 10—in the backseat, which is also odd. (And no, a head-on crash would not have thrown him back there.) The car's windshield didn't break, so I have no idea where the kid got all those facial lacerations… not to mention the cut to his jugular. As I said, the accident set-up was just strange.

Oh well, I can chalk that up to dramatic license and take it for what it is: an opportunity for our guys to do their best in a bad situation. Johnny makes a leg splint out of a map book or whatever that large magazine-like thing is. And Chet pitches in however he can; he proves to be very handy and useful in a crisis (thank you, firefighter training!). I still don't understand, though, why Chet didn't hop in the Land Rover and drive up ahead looking for some help.

Anyway, they eventually find themselves riding in a multipurpose hearse/ambulance and get taken to Middleville Community Hospital, which is aptly named as the community is in the "middle" of nowhere. They encounter a protesting nurse and both Johnny and Roy have to use their Serious voices in order to get their point across. But it's the arrival of Doctor Frick that saves the day. The unconventional doc looks like a Woodstock holdover: long hair, a big 'stache that Chet would envy, jeans, and an old denim work shirt on top of what looks like a poorly tie-dyed undershirt (Imagine him and Kel Brackett standing next to each other... boggles the mind!) In any case, he does a "fine job of vascular surgery," and Johnny admits that Frick's appearance really "blows his mind."

All this excitement was pretty interesting to the three firefighters involved, but the guys at Station 51 are singularly unimpressed (except maybe Cap). But there's no time to discuss it further because the tones go off and we get the car-over-a-cliff call that will lead to Johnny's no-good, very-bad day. I think I mentioned last time the tractor driver's amazing magic helmet, with the disappearing and reappearing face shield. That's just too funny. I also liked seeing the engine fill up Copter 14 so it could do a water drop. (Random thought: where does Stoker take Big Red to refill her?)

Back to the crashed car: the FFs finally reach the victims by following the reluctant dozer driver. There are three victims—those crazy teenagers, always speeding and racing their cars! With the help of the other guys, and the guys from Engine 85, Roy and Johnny treat the victims and they're all transported topside. Now, this is where logic gets a little fuzzy again. First flaw in the story is that with three victims, I really think *both* paramedics would have gone in the chopper with them. One paramedic can deal with two victims, but with three, I think both should have gone. However… this being a TV show and the writers wanting to torture their audience and create some high drama, that doesn't happen. Roy goes in the chopper by himself, leaving Johnny at the scene.

Cap calls in to LA that the engine is available at scene and they're all preparing to leave, when of course Johnny realizes that he left the HT down at the accident site. He goes to retrieve it and we all know what happens next. Cap contacts LA again and says "we're *not* available." Also, even though we've never seen or heard it before, and never see/hear it again, it's shown that the "paramedic bitten by rattlesnake" announcement has been received at Rampart's base station. At the scene, Chet and Marco are dispatched down to where Johnny is, and the two of them help him get on the tractor for the ride back to the top. He's placed on the top of the engine (when did Mike drive it back down there?) and thus begins one of some fans' favorite scenes. Which, unfortunately, I have to call into question.

The other FFs are perfectly qualified to take a victim's pulse, respiration, and even BP (we've seen them do it before), so there really was no need for Johnny to do it all himself. But to me, the biggest goof here is about the IV. And why is it a goof? Because *Roy would have taken the drug box with him.* In fact, we can see the chopper co-pilot carrying the drug box as they're getting ready to load up Copter 14. So in real life, the paramedic wouldn't have been able to start an IV on himself because he would not have an IV available. But again, this being a TV show, a drug box magically appears and *¡voila!* we have a dramatic scene.

Long story short, tense moments ensue, engine screams across the county on the way to Rampart General, and a deathly-pale John Gage is wheeled into a treatment room. All the station guys are hanging around in the hallway but Chet joins Roy in the treatment room and seems reluctant to leave. This is the "full circle" I referenced earlier: Chet and Johnny and their never-ending pretend-antagonism toward each other. Of course it's just a smokescreen for caring on both sides, grudging and unacknowledged as it may be. One's concerned when the other is hurt. Chet goes along with Roy to visit John in the hospital, and in return Gage shares his home-baked cookies with his sort-of-but-not-really nemesis Chet.

3.7 The Promotion

Agreed, that was the hokiest depiction of an accident (heavy smog with chain-reaction pileup on a highway) this show has ever done. (And I give the show credit that usually all traffic accidents look much more realistic than this.) Even before they get to the pile-up, as they're leaving the station, there's some sort of bad "fog filter" over what is probably just a stock shot of the engine and squad pulling out.

At that accident scene, Roy encounters a man who's worried about his brother, stuck in a crashed car. Roy tells the brother to "close the hood" of his car to snuff out the fire, then he discovers the other brother is dead. Then, when Marco and Chet arrive, they automatically open the hood to put out the flames with an extinguisher. Is that an automatic procedure at accidents? I've seen Chet do it once or twice in other eps (including Snake Bite), but in this case I didn't see them do it to any other vehicles as they passed. Also, there weren't any flames showing on this car before they opened it, and Roy didn't tell them to check it, either.

Again we have a child actor--in this case, a *very* young one-- who did a very good job. She looked positively lifeless when being carried out of the vehicle, and stayed immobile as Chet did CPR (and "mouth-to-mouth" with her cheek, if you'll notice). I wonder how they got the child at that young age to be so still for so long?

Funny, though, when Roy was dealing with the mother (possible spine injury), she told him she couldn't move, and he said "stay right there." Ha ha, no problem, since I can't move anyway! But I love it when I hear the paramedics say "don't do anything, let us do all the work." For some reason that sounds so... efficient, and professional. And realistic, too.

Anyway, wrapped around the chain-reaction accident, and a second pool-dunking for Roy, this was another of the Big Issues episodes. And of course I liked it, I like the soul-searching and heart-felt conversations as Roy considers taking a promotion that would take him away from his paramedic duties. I really like that Roy asks Brackett (and Early) their opinions, as it shows how much he respects them.

Also, I liked the final rescue, with Johnny having a hurt leg and Roy literally being blown out a window onto the ladder. Lots of opportunities to see our guys in turnout coats, air-packs, masks, helmets, etc. And them coming down the ladder.... whoo, ultimate action and coolness. I've heard from those who've trained in firefighting, that that little "flip" Roy did off the ladder is something they actually practice for when they have to go out a window head-first. (By the way, did anyone notice that at least twice after they landed, Roy put his hand on Johnny's leg? I'll refrain from commenting further.) I'm sure those might have been stunt-guys on the ladder (especially as stand-in for Roy, going head-first like that) but I still love that scene!!!

~ ~ ~

An Issues Episode, at least for one of our fave paramedics. Roy does very well on the Engineer's exam (big surprise!) and is eligible for a promotion to engineer when a slot becomes available, which, of course, means more money. That's the good news. The bad news is... he'd have to take a promotion to engineer and stop being a paramedic. It's an either/or situation: he can *either* be a paramedic, which is paid at the lowest rate in the department, *or* he can become an engineer and trade earning more money for doing something he loves to do. Quite a dilemma, and it weighs on him. Johnny alternately encourages his friend to grab the brass ring, and take *him* and *his* welfare into consideration in making the decision. (But only jokingly, of course.)

Meanwhile, Station 51 is called to a fog-induced chain reaction accident on some big freeway which involves dozens of vehicles. In addition to the fake fog, I noticed that yet again the small child who's trapped in the wreck is only seen as a pair of shoes/feet buried under something. Or, in this case, some*one*. In that earlier episode, with "Debbie!!", wasn't it only her shoes that were visible in the drunk-driving wreck? And the small boy who went into the burning house after his dog and hid under the bed in the other Roy-centric episode? Again, we saw only his shoes under the bed. (Speaking of car wrecks, why are these young victims usually little girls?? Even in the episode in which Brackett was involved in an accident, the other victim was a girl.)

I fast-forwarded through the "suicide" call. Same with Joel and the heart problem at Rampart. The only redeeming quality of these scenes is that we get to see Roy take another dip in the drink, that is, fall into a swimming pool. And afterward there's a touching scene of Roy taking a moment to get acquainted with the engine, once he decides to take the promotion. (I bet Stoker secretly followed right after him, wiping Roy's fingerprints off Mike's beloved Big Red.)

One thing I have a quibble with regarding the final rescue: I know the engineers generally stick with the engine at the scene (duh!) and that's fine and important, but on the other hand, you don't have to be a paramedic to search a building for a missing person. Again, the most highly-trained members of the team are the *only* ones who can run into the burning building to save someone?? Doesn't make a lot of sense to me.

The final call, and resulting rescue, is one of my all-time favorites. Johnny goes into a burning building to find the requisite "someone left inside," with Roy holding the lifeline. Explosion occurs, Johnny falls, Roy can't get an answer from him, and also can't get Cap's attention. So he goes in after his partner. Roy finds Johnny, who's got a hurt leg or something. They can't get out the way they came in so they have to go to the 2nd floor, but the fire is creeping around them. Roy takes charge and gets things taken care of, even as the fire (and the room they're in) is about to flash over. The other FFs get a ladder up to the window and the security guard is handed over to safety. Johnny starts limping down the ladder and is about halfway to the bottom when the fire finally goes *boom!*, blowing Roy right out the window and down the ladder. I love watching that scene, with him falling right on top of Johnny, who tries to catch him, and they both fall over to the ground. (By the way, I know that's not really Kevin and Randy doing that, but I'm pretending here, so don't ruin it for me, a'ight?) Anyway, I think that's one of my favorite scenes in the whole series. Roy must have enjoyed the experience, too, as he then tells Johnny that decided to turn down the promotion and try again next year, when maybe the rules will be changed. Too bad they didn't revisit the issue again at some point, if not with another promotion episode (too repetitive), then at least some sort of conversation about it.

But yes, another good Issues episode. Or perhaps not really issues, but more like a dilemma.

3.8 Insomnia

...ZZZZZZZZZ

(Or, Johnny wants attention. No, he doesn't want attention. Wait, yes, he does.) Ha-ha, yeah, just kidding, not ragging on Fireman Gage for real, don'tchaknow.

Anyhoo, that sentiment is somewhat justified. First he doesn't want anyone but Roy to know what's going on with his lack of sleep. Then he gets ticked that Chet found out that he (Johnny) can't get to sleep. Then he practically baits the other guys into asking him about it, but then later he doesn't like it when they *do* show an interest. They even make him a stokes cradle. Or perhaps I should say stokes hammock.

Before I finish that topic, here's the "other" stuff of this episode.

~ First scene in the dorm, there's a little ledge/shelf between Roy and John's bunk. I don't think it was there in earlier seasons. And there's even a book on it.

~ Have we ever seen anyone at the station use a saucer with their coffee cups? In this ep Johnny does it twice. It's almost more of a bowl than a saucer, looks kinda strange to me.

~ First call (exploding boat) comes in at 7:05, but based on what we see during the drive to the scene and at the scene, it was more like late morning or early afternoon.

~ In this rescue, pause or slo-mo the scene as the ambulance arrives and passes right in front of the camera. In the back window of the ambulance, you can clearly see reflection of studio lights, people, reflectors, even an aluminum ladder (I think). Good thing nobody could have seen it 40 years ago.

~ Re the pot-smoking computer guy, after Johnny inserts the esophageal airway and Roy hands him the thing for it, you can see Johnny's watch. Looks like it says 1:00, maybe? Or possibly 6:00, I couldn't say for sure since I don't know how big the hour/minute hands were.

~ The guy pinned in by the truck--from his first comment or two, I wouldn't have automatically categorized it as "euphoria." To me it would have sounded just like he was trying not to panic, trying to keep the mood light, etc. Now, if he'd laughed uncontrollably, that would have been more of a tip-off, but it could have been taken as him simply making light of a bad situation. Good thing the writers knew better.

~ Speaking of the Marijuana Man and his co-worker... weren't either of them worried about their jobs? Being caught smoking weed on the job--not the best career move!!

~ When Roy went into the stone pit at the quarry, I guess he wasn't worried about slipping into the hole like the man did? Also, as they were going into the shaft for the boy, Cap said "we'll set up your stuff out here," and Johnny said "OK, you do that." To me the way Johnny/Randy said that sounded odd, as if it was an unscripted comment, or maybe he was just tired or bored and not really at the top of his game at that moment. Did that strike anyone else as odd?

~ Lastly, with that same rescue, how did they know when to stop the conveyor belt thing? Nothing was showing, and it took an extra 5-8 seconds from the time they said "stop" to when it actually stopped, and it's not like the boy's legs were dangling down or anything. Or did they just think they'd freed up enough stones to be able to reach him by feel? (Again, I guess the writers knew better.) I know, it doesn't really matter, the important thing is they *did* know when to have the belt turned off, and they *did* get the boy out. Happy endings all around.

Two more things:

1) Love the scene with Roy coming into the kitchen while Johnny was making the cocoa. Hot bunker-pants alert!!!

But, one thing I've noticed before... Johnny seems to wear the standard V-neck t-shirt. But Roy's shirt has a neck with a deeper "v" cut. Not that I'm complaining, as it gives a peak at his alluring chest-fur. But it's odd that the two t-shirts seem to be quite different. This isn't the first or only time that I've noticed Roy's shirt being deeper-cut. It's just quite obvious here, with them standing side-by-side.

2) I know the final scene was filmed for comic relief, but it does sort of bother me that it was written that way, with Johnny clinging half-asleep to the back of the engine as it rolls out on a call in the middle of the night. Obviously Roy would *not* have just turned off the light in the dorm and gone back to bed. He would have contacted Cap right away* to let him know that Johnny was on the tailboard. Dangerous enough during the day, it could be positively fatal at night, especially when the person in question is half-asleep. Also, what if the squad got called out on a run--what would Roy do, go out alone?? Ha, of course not.

* I wonder if he would have to go through dispatch ("LA") to contact the engine? Even if they keep another set of HTs at the station, the engine would be out of range before Roy could even try.

~ ~ ~

I liked almost everything about this episode. The rescues weren't particularly exciting but they were different and interesting. The boat explosion at a traffic intersection, the weed-crazed computer nerd, and the man pinned by the truck, etc. All just a little different and not the standard heart attack or factory fire with "there's still one person left inside!"

From earlier thread: About the guy pinned by the truck--from his first comment or two, I wouldn't have automatically suspected "euphoria." To me it would have sounded just like he was trying not to panic, trying to keep the mood light, etc. Also, he didn't look like he was pinned that tightly... at all. Certainly not tightly enough to serve as a tourniquet. But I guess they couldn't exactly film it to look like he was practically being cut in half. Not back then, at least.

Also, last time I discussed the gravel-pit rescue I wondered how Johnny knew (or guessed, or whatever) when to turn the machine off. Good thing it wasn't extremely time-sensitive, as it took about 5-10 seconds to get things shut down. But how did he know when--or if--the kid was accessible?

About the insomnia storyline... at first Johnny didn't want the other guys to know about it because they'd rag on him. Later he practically baited them to comment on his plight. (Which, perversely, they didn't.) But then when they finally do acknowledge it, he's not happy with that either, so I don't really know what he wanted.

And yeah, the final scene was totally unrealistic. As if Roy would just let Johnny hang onto the engine while he's half-asleep and not do anything about it. It made for a funny scene, but it's *not* what would have happened.

* * *

About the dad who'd been in an accident with his son... yeah, at first I thought he was gonna be one of those selfish parents that says "Hey, I'm the one you need to look at, never mind the kid." But I think--or have the impression--that he saw the kid had no obvious injuries like bleeding or bruising or broken bones, so he assumed the boy was okay. Plus, if he asked the kid, I'm sure he would've said he was fine, so maybe (I'm hoping, at least) that's why it never occurred to him that his son was injured. But I do think it was touching that after Brackett mentioned the skull fracture and recommended a skull series or whatever, and then said they'd take an x-ray of the dad's arm, the dad had pretty much forgotten about his own minor boo-boo and was totally concerned about his son. Now *that* is what a parent would do. Better late than never, I guess.

3.9 Inheritance Tax

(Also known as The Episode in Which Johnny Loses the Side Part.) Yes, it's the first time we see the "new" John Gage hair, *without* the LACoFD-approved side part. He's moving into his best hair look: not too long (yet), not too short, could still use some judicious snipping, but overall, a good look for him. Add the fact that Roy's hair has looked good for a number of (or most) eps in S3, and we have a very pretty pair, indeed.

First off, in the first rescue, did anyone notice that we don't really "see" any of the Engine 51 guys? The engine arrives, we *barely* get a glimpse of Cap in the cab (but only if you pause it), and can identify Chet in the jumpseat behind him, but oddly enough, none of them get out of the engine or even speak. At least, not that we see. This sort of ties in to a theory I have about this show.

Moving on..... The paramedics get called by good ol' "Mrs. C" to treat her boss, Mr. Wheeler-Dealer. (This was just before Marion Ross appeared in Happy Days, I believe.)   And Wheeler-Dealer was sedated and put in the CCU. Man, that didn't look like any CCU unit *I* ever saw. To me it looked like a semi-private room with a few extra machines included.

So Roy and John are heirs, eh? In the scene in which they're working on the squad, after closing the hood, watch for the disappearing oil can. Johnny's holding the can. No, his hands are empty. Yep, there's the can again. More TV magic!

Speaking of the inheritance, it's so funny to see Johnny squirm while the lawyer looks at his papers and hems-and-haws before getting down to the subject at hand. (Roy, meanwhile, is his usual taciturn self.) And then of course the tones sound, no doubt frustrating Gage further. (Although he's at least distracted, I guess.)

I liked some things about this structure fire. For one thing, there wasn't the usual "Wait, where's Harry? Oh no, he's still inside!" at the last minute, necessitating our boys to go in search of said lost person. For another thing, I noticed that even a Captain was getting in on the action with the fire. Not Cap Stanley, but another one... although Cap Stanley definitely pulls his weight when necessary too. Still, nice to see that captains are willing to pitch in to get the job done. (Especially with the Battalion Chief there, --big surprise to see everyone pitching in, right?)

At the end of the fire scene, when the victim is being loaded into the ambulance, Johnny says "Cap released me for hospital follow-up." Um, what is that all about??? Roy rode in the ambulance with the victim, which doesn't require any approval from Cap. Does Johnny mean that Cap said he didn't have to stay and do 'clean-up' with the other FFs? The paramedics don't usually do that when they have a victim... they're automatically both cleared to go to Rampart. Or so I always assumed.

I just rewatched the fire and noticed something odd. At about 36:50 mark (on Netflix), right after the man-on-fire is hosed down and Roy climbs up to get him, the scene/footage changes suddenly; for about 1-2 seconds it looks like a different piece of film was spliced in--same location, but the background is just a bit different, and also, the fire is gone, so those split seconds are darker than the others. Then the "real" scene resumes. I bet they just had to re-shoot that one segment for some reason to bridge the parts around it, and it's so quick it mostly goes unnoticed. (An amateur guess.)

At Rampart, Wheeler-Dealer man is looking at a magazine, and one page of the magazine has a large headline or tagline that says "Mommy Forgot." I wonder what that was all about?? An ad? If so, for what? Or maybe an article.

Lastly, I hope Roy and John didn't spend their $18.75 inheritance all in one place.

~ ~ ~

I like this episode, although it has a couple of forgettable weak spots. But for the most part it's a keeper.

The *big* news of this episode is that~~ ta-da ~~ Johnny's officially done with the LACoFD haircut. This is where Pretty Johnny is born—hallelujah!!

We start off with Squad 51 already on the road, which is unusual in itself. But it was apparently done for two reasons. 1) The squad had to beat the engine to the scene so Johnny could have the chance to be creative with the car and the power lines. And 2) No spoken lines by anyone on the engine was a money-saver for the producers; as it was, no faces are clearly seen, although Cap and Chet can be glimpsed in a blink-and-you-miss-it drive-by. Also, this scene another version of the Debbie Syndrome... this one consists of "Billy, stay in the car!" Seriously, I half expected the kid to open the door and say "What? What do you want?? Why are you yelling to me??"

Back at the station, Roy tells Johnny the news of their bequest from the RMV— Rich Mystery Victim. At that point they don't know anything other than she "remembered" them in her will. Of course, Gage takes that inch and stretches it to his usual mile, calculating the value of her three-story house, pool, and tennis courts. Good thing his hair hasn't grown that much, since he has enough trouble seeing with those dollar signs in his eyes.

Speaking of money, their next call is to a wheeler-dealer who wants to postpone his heart attack 'til he can take care of some lucrative trades. Needless to say, our no-nonsense paramedics get him to Rampart despite his objections. Later Mrs. Cunningham tells Brackett that Winthrop is really a nice guy underneath all his greed. (By the way, should Brackett have been discussing Winthrop's condition with her, since she's not related in any way?)

Back at Rampart, Joe Early is treating the most adorable patients *ever*. Steve is cute as a button and at first I always think he has a gumball in his cheeks, but that's just how his pinch-worthy cheeks look, apparently. Pete is the quiet one with the unruly hair and boo-boo on his leg. They get a kick out of hearing each other's heartbeats; maybe when they come back in a few days they'll be ready to try a full skull series and a spinal tap.

While the engine is gone, John and Roy work on the squad (really? how much work does it need, anyway?) and we learn that Roy dreams of having some alone time [*cough*no wife*cough] and Johnny thinks he's "young enough" to handle two girls at once. Nothing like a little menage-a-Gage to get the imagination working, eh?? From there we get a call to treat the boring hamburger-eating contest loser. Meanwhile, other than Chet, we haven't officially seen anyone else from the station yet. Like I said, Mark VII trying to control actor costs, maybe..??

When we do finally see Cap, Marco, and Mike, and they're allowed to actually talk, Roy and Johnny tell them about their impending windfall. Roy tries to reassure everyone that nothing's changed and they're still just "one of the guys," but Chet is not-so-subtly hinting that maybe some of their newfound riches could be put toward updating the station. Who knows, maybe that could be considered charity??

The final big rescue is at one of the dozens of paint factories that apparently litter LA County. It's nothing too exciting, but it did give Dennis Donnelly a chance to get creative with his filming and there was an impressive display of fire equipment on scene.

Which brings us back to the inheritance. It's so friggin' funny watching Johnny during the first lawyer scene. He's like a four-year-old and literally can't keep from squirming in his chair. In the second lawyer scene he's about to lean into the lawyer's lap, he's so anxious for the man to get to the point. But by the time all the different "deductions" are read, he's sitting back with his hand over his eyes, regretting having told the other guys anything about this. Why does he never learn???

Fun facts:

~ $1,211,000 back in 1973 would be about $6.4 million today. Not a bad piece of change.

~ Their final payout of $18.75 calculates to about $100 in 2014 money. Maybe they can pool their money and rent a boat. Johnny can bring a Playboy magazine in lieu of a "couple of girls."

~ Stock footage has been sloppy lately. Showing two attendants in the front seat of the ambulance on the way to the hospital, and also the guys magically wearing their blue jackets as they leave Rampart in the squad.

~ Okay, Winthrop in the CCU... that was unlike any CCU I ever saw, or probably ever existed. It looked like a normal private room. My mother was in an ICU ward around the same time as this show and it was an actual ward, with multiple patients where staff could keep an eye on them. Privacy was not an issue, much less the patients having telephones.

~ It seems the only magazines that patients get to read at Rampart are medical journals, as evidenced by the pharmaceutical ads we see. (However this doesn't apply to Dr. Early, who apparently has access to a secret stash of skin mags.)

3.10 Zero

I wonder why this ep is titled Zero? No obvious reason that I can see. Anyway, this ep had a brief guest-turn by JoAnn Worley as a screamer. (And no, not the fun kind, at least, not that we see.) I thought the audio sync-ing was kind of 'off' for her on this scene, but maybe it was just Netflix. Also, when she was passing by on her bike, Roy got Johnny's attention in kind of a strange way... he seemed to poke his butt. Or maybe he pinched it, I don't know. Either way, afterward they probably both had a cigarette and went on with their day. But I did wonder... since their shifts are 24 hours, and usually begin and end at 8am (or thereabouts), why did they change from bunker gear to uniforms? That call should have been either at the end of a shift (early a.m.) or the beginning of one.

At the scene of the kid on a building ledge, when J and R first arrive, the captain says "DeSoto, you go up the aerial ladder. Gage, you follow and block." Then fade to intro. A minute or so later, once the ladder is extended, we hear the cap again say

"DeSoto, you go up the aerial." It's the same audio clip we heard earlier, edited for brevity. And we hear Roy say "Okay, Cap," although I'm not convinced that wasn't added in later too, as I think he really said "Okay, [something else]." Anyway, once they were up on the ladder and talking to the kid, did anyone else kind of worry every time Roy turned to see what the boy was looking at, looking at that other building, etc? The kid could have taken that opportunity of him looking away to make his move off the building. Yikes.

Other than the depressing topic (an 8-year-old contemplating suicide, as well as child abuse) one thing that I don't like about this episode is Mariette Hartley. I hesitate to say that I don't like her, because honestly, she's actually very good in this episode, and she's a good actress. But I think I shy away from her because I often don't like the characters she plays. Anyway, I did think it odd that, at Rampart, after the boy Tommy physically flinched in fear when she came into the room, the doctors then allowed her in to see Tommy... *alone*. Without asking the kid if he'd be OK with it, or even giving him a head's-up that she was coming in. I found that a little insensitive for a show that can sometimes be overly sensitive. (Oh, and we had the soap-opera music again. Ugh.)

But one of the big storylines of this episode was Johnny freezing in front of news cameras, particularly in an interview the paramedics did and which was watched by the whole station. I was a little baffled by some of this, and feel like I need a flow chart to follow it properly. First Johnny accuses Roy of 'horning in' on him during the interview--and he says it in front of Dixie, too. Then in the squad Johnny does *not* blame Roy at all; instead he's bummed and worried about the other guys teasing him, but Roy says "I cut you off before you could form your thoughts." So not only is Roy now agreeing with Johnny's earlier (false) comment, but he's also using it to give Johnny an 'out' in front of the others. Sort of like a big brother allowing the younger one to "blame me if you want to." But Johnny said he wanted to do it *his* way. And yeah, his way of dealing with the guys was pretty darn good. Clever and effective--bearding the lion in its den, so to speak. And you could tell that Roy was pleased (and surprised?) by it, as well. But then of course Johnny did *not* get over his camera-paralysis and he choked again, at the fire. This time Roy seemed very comfortable taking over. (Even though the boy they had rescued seemed to move magically from one shot to the next.)

~ ~ ~

I'm at a loss as to the title of this one... "zero" seems to have nothing to do with anything in the episode. Except maybe that's what the little boy Tommy felt with his empty eyes...???

Anyhoo....

The ep opens with the squad racing to some warehouse, apparently in the early morning, since the guys are in their bunker pants sans uniform shirts. (*fans self*) The situation is... the woman is a screamer. For therapeutic reasons, of course. I believe--although I can't recall if it was mentioned here or elsewhere--that the JoAnn Worley scene was originally filmed for another episode. Makes me wonder how often they "shuffled" these standalone scenes, tossing one in here and there when needed. In any case, this makes two eps in a row that didn't open at the station.

As much as we all love Johnny's new 'do (and the arrival of Pretty Johnny), now it makes some of the stock footage out of date, as we see side-parted Johnny getting into the squad a couple of times in this episode, including the first run which is called out while everyone is watching the interview. The guys and Truck 85 are called to a kid-on-ledge call. Roy is tapped to go up as point-man and Johnny backing him. We see Roy being all soothing and gentle with little Tommy, even while ungrammatically saying "don't it" as he makes small talk with the kid. Unfortunately, Tommy not only moves away from Roy, he then decides he'd rather take the quick way down, and steps off the ledge. Luckily Roy is pretty quick himself and catches the kid. Although it confused me... for one thing, Roy continued to talk soothingly to Tommy, as if Tommy was afraid, and for another thing, didn't it occur to Roy that the kid might fight him and try to get away (and, again, *down*)?

Anyway, in general I don't like the Mariette Hartley story... one minute the kid recoils from her, and ten minutes later, after she confessed to hitting him (!!!), the doctors allow her in the room with him.... *alone.* Whiskey tango foxtrot!! I seem to remember another episode with an abused kid, and while we're all supposed to think the dad is the culprit, it (again) turns out to be the mom. Except the sharp doctors ask her if she'd been in an accident or suffered a head injury or something, which conveniently explained the behavior *without* making her into a bad guy. Apparently Mrs. Mannering doesn't rate that kind of consideration; instead her situation is 'explained' by extreme stress. Because after all, the mom can't possibly be just plain bad.

By the way, not sure why Johnny rode in the ambulance with the kid, after Tommy and Roy had that whole "how many antennas" history going for them. You'd think Roy would have been the one.

Still sticking with this storyline, I had to laugh when Dixie told the mother that Tommy was in X-ray. We saw the orderly go in to get Tommy to take him to X-ray, but we never saw him come back out. So technically, Tommy was still in the treatment room and not in X-ray. In any case, we got the schmaltzy, soapy music in this ep. One thing we did *not* get was one of Dixie's coffee-laden heart-to-hearts.

The other minor rescue in this ep was the donut-guy who got stuck in the machinery, which was light-hearted and non-dramatic, but it did give Johnny (Randy) the opportunity to eat yet again. Other than this, the main paramedic/station action was Johnny realizing he had to live down his on-camera meltdown. He told Roy he'd handle it and, while willingly taking the blame on himself for 'stealing' Johnny's spotlight, Roy agrees that's the best plan: let Johnny handle it. And he did... quite well, actually. I was proud of him. And so was Roy, apparently.

The final action was yet another warehouse fire, and--surprise, surprise!--someone was stuck inside. Bigger surprise: it's a kid!! Seriously, what's up with these LA County parents that their kids are constantly wandering where they don't belong, setting fires, drinking from strange bottles, etc. What's up with that?? Anyway, I thought Roy sounded like he was out of breath pretty much every time we heard him talk in this one. Even in the post-fire interview... which he again commandeered from his partner. (Not that Johnny minded, but I'm just sayin'.) Yeah, Roy sounded like he was out of breath both inside and outside the building. And with the TV reporter, Johnny apparently decided to cut his losses and make a quiet exit, leaving Roy to it. By the way, I wonder if there is/was any policy about firefighters talking to the press at the scene of an incident. I should think there would be; that should be the purview of the highest-ranking officer at the scene (or communications officer, if one is present).

3.11 The Promise

So, The Promise.... At the automotive garage, Cap sent our paramedics out to "check the rest of the area." Why did he do that? The obvious problem was the car on fire, and it wasn't until the owner wondered where the guy was who'd been fixing that car that we had the first clue that someone might be missing. So why did Cap automatically send the boys out to search around? Dramatic license, I guess; there are times when it obviously trumps logic when it comes to TV. And why did Johnny give the victim's age as "approximately 26"? Usually people approximate things in round numbers: 20, 25, 30, etc. How does 26 look so different from 25??

Someone mentioned the interesting directorial views in the previous episode, and we saw quite a bit of that again in The Promise, with the camera being the patient and Brackett examining "him" up close and personal. I have to say, I'm not a fan of that type of shot. I find it awkward and almost uncomfortable. (Don't know why.)

So Roy is friends with a nurse named Ann. How could that possibly be news to Johnny? Roy mentioned getting coffee with Ann occasionally... where is the intrepid Mr. Gage when this happens? It can't only happen when Roy works other shifts, or when Johnny is out sick or something. I call bogus on Roy apparently getting to know this woman to such a degree that they can "confide" in each other* without Johnny having the least clue. Again.... dramatic license. (But I did like the scene in the squad when Johnny was mad and the radio beeped. He grabbed up the radio and barked "Squad 51" in sort of a disgusted tone. That was funny, and pretty realistic, I thought.)

Later, we get a scene that supposedly takes place first thing on their shift-- Mike raises the flag, and Roy greets Johnny with "Good morning" and asks about the day off. But 2 minutes later when Johnny is in Cap's office, the time is 10:40 (and the call they get is dispatched at 10:42). Gee, who knew shifts started at 10:30 am??

Joe Early goes up to Brackett in the hallway and asks about the catatonic guy from the auto garage. Brackett says "let's go check on him." Lo and behold, they turn down a hallway and there's his room... on the SIXTH floor. Here I thought they were standing at the base station in the ED (ground floor), but nooooo, they were inexplicably on the sixth floor. They really *must* be the only doctors in that hospital.

Final rescue of catatonic man, after he freaks out and jumps out the window at Rampart... did anyone else notice that Roy was *NOT* tied off when he got on that ledge? He was in real danger of splatting on the pavement if that guy shoved him. Bad planning on someone's part! Also, after they got the guy subdued and sent him down on the snorkel, Johnny unhooked himself from the rope he'd been on. Maybe he figured if Roy wasn't secured, he wouldn't be either. (And why they didn't just climb back in through the window instead of making the snorkel come back up to get them... who knows!!) Also as they were talking to Brackett on the ground, the snorkel truck rolled past. Guess they got the snorkel back in place and undid all the counter-balance thingies, etc., in record time--mere seconds! Either that or it was just the magic of how time passes on TV.

*On one hand, I'm not sure what Roy would 'confide' to his "friend" Ann that he couldn't or wouldn't tell to his wife. On the other hand, why did Johnny say "I wouldn't feel right" about asking Ann out, and that he "wouldn't want to get in the way." Just what exactly did he think was going on that he would "get in the way" of?? That didn't make a lot of sense to me. On the other hand, it almost looked like he was teasing when he said that. At least, up until he learned that Roy had Ann over to dinner and didn't invite *him*.

~ ~ ~

Much of this is cut and pasted from last time, since I noticed these same things again this time, so comments might be the same. Plus a few original things. Wait, that might not be a *good* thing....

We know the "promise" of the title is Paula's promise (from first season's Mascot) to Johnny to get him a puppy. Thing is, I don't think he remembered such a promise. So yeah, it doesn't work out all that great for Fireman Gage. He doesn't even get a date with Paula, as far as I could see. (Doesn't work out all that great for Sam, either, probably.)

At the service station for the first call, Cap sent our paramedics out to "check the rest of the area." Why did he do that? The obvious problem was the car on fire (duh), and it wasn't until the owner wondered where the guy was who'd been fixing that car that we had the first clue that someone might be missing. So why did Cap automatically send the boys out to search around? He's never done that before. Dramatic license, I guess; it obviously trumps logic when it comes to TV.

So Roy is friends with a nurse named Ann. How could Johnny not know that? Roy mentioned getting coffee with Ann occasionally... where is the intrepid Mr. Gage when this happens? It can't *only* happen when Roy works other shifts, or when Johnny is out sick or whatever. I call bogus on Roy apparently getting to know this woman to such a degree that they can "confide" in each other* without Johnny having the least clue. Again.... dramatic license. (But I did like the scene in the squad when Johnny was mad and the radio beeped. He grabbed up the radio and barked "Squad 51" in sort of a disgusted tone. That was funny, and pretty realistic, I thought.)

Later, we get a scene that supposedly takes place first thing on their shift-- Mike raises the flag, and Roy greets Johnny with "Good morning" and asks about the day off. But 2 minutes later when Johnny is in Cap's office, the time is 10:40 (and the

211

call they get is dispatched at 10:42). Gee, who knew shifts started at 10:30 am??

Joe Early goes up to Brackett in the hallway and asks about the catatonic guy. Brackett says "let's go check on him." Lo and behold, they turn down a hallway and there's his room... on the SIXTH floor. Here I thought they were standing at the base station in the ED (ground floor), but nooooo, the two Emergency doctors were apparently on the sixth floor treating patients. They really *must* be the only doctors in that hospital.

Final rescue of catatonic man... for some reason Roy did NOT secure himself to anything before he got on that ledge. What's up with that?? He was in real danger of splatting on the pavement if that guy shoved him. Also, after they got the guy subdued and sent him down on the snorkel, why they didn't just climb back in through the window instead of making the snorkel come back up?? Lastly, as the paramedics were talking to Brackett on the ground, the snorkel bucket was plainly visible behind them. Then they walked to the squad and as soon as they got in, the snorkel rolled past in the background. Guess 127s got the snorkel back in place and undid all the counter-balance thingies, etc., in record time-- mere seconds! Either that or it was just the magic of how time passes on TV.

*On one hand, I'm not sure what Roy would "confide" to his friend Ann that he couldn't or wouldn't tell to his wife--or Johnny, for that matter. On the other hand, why did Johnny say "I wouldn't feel right" about asking Ann out, and that he "wouldn't want to get in the way." Just what exactly did he think was going on that he would "get in the way" of?? That didn't make a lot of sense to me. On the third hand, it almost looked like he was teasing when he said that. At least, up until he learned that Roy had Ann over to dinner and didn't invite him.

This'n'that:

~ The garage owner's name was Roy. Guess the writers finally figured out they use the name Charlie too often. (So what do they do? Use another duplicate name. Duh!)

~ Chet was studying again... apparently he's getting a head start on the next engineer's exam, so maybe he'll do better than 74th.

~ Speaking of Chet, he's antagonistic toward Boot, but seems to get along with Sam, and later he'll positively dote on Henry. What's his problem with Boot???

~ The blue jackets were back. No badges/pins on them this time, though.

~ The ashtray was visible on the desk at Rampart's base station. Also, they used a glass IV bottle on Catatonic Man. I thought they'd done away with them by this time.

*   *   *

> "She confides in me and I confide in her and we're
> friends." Uhhhh, I know there are situations where that is
> fine, but for Roy it just seemed odd.

Yeah, I have to wonder what the writer was doing with this storyline. I have no problem with Roy being friendly with a nurse or even inviting her to join him and his wife for dinner (although I imagine JoAnne would have wanted to fix the girl up, stat, to make sure she was 'safe,' knowwhatImean?) But the whole "confiding" thing was definitely over the top. Totally out of character for Roy.

But the more I think of it, and think of the other episode where Roy has a not-so-secret admirer (and again in some ways acts OOC), I believe that these two stories aren't really about Roy at all. They're about Johnny. As far as Gage is concerned, Roy is pretty much a dull, one-dimensional married man, so he can't wrap his head around the fact that a woman actually finds Roy appealing. Johnny's also flummoxed to learn that Roy has friends *other than him*, and--even more surprising-- one of these friends is an attractive woman. In both instances Johnny comes across a situation that seems inconceivable to him. Unfortunately, no matter why it was done, I don't think Johnny comes off looking very good.

3.12 Body Language

My subtitle for this one would be: "Roy gets an admirer, Johnny (almost) gets a wife."

And given the circumstances where that redneck rodeo guy is concerned, I think it's more a matter of Forrest Gump sounding like the hillbilly horse-rider, rather than the opposite.

- At the hospital, a kid tries to trade his walker for a pair of crutches. Query: has anyone ever seen a kid using a walker? I mean a kid with a broken leg, that is. I never have. I think he was right to think his friends would pick on him. Unfortunately.

- Crop-duster pilot... at the hospital it looked like there was a tube sticking out of his chest/lung/torso. I assume that was the prescribed treatment for pneumothorax, but as is often the case on this show, things are done without being explained. This isn't a criticism of that, I'd rather it be that way than otherwise; just an observation.

~ "A host of golden daffodils...." The mantra of Bobby's daughter—er, I mean, some flaky girl named Pam. (She is very pretty, though; and she appeared quite often on E! and Adam-12.) But her character in this one seems to take a shine to Roy, both at the park and at the hospital. When he and Johnny are getting ready to leave the treatment room, Pam says dreamily "You take care too, Roy." This sort of catches Johnny's attention and he looks at the doctors and sort of shrugs. (Poor Johnny; he still has girl trouble--although not the usual kind this time--and girls are *still* falling for Roy.)

~ At the rescue of Cowboy Tex, Roy got on the biophone to Rampart while Johnny checks for broken bones, but as soon as Rampart responds, Johnny says "I'll get it, I'll get it." That seemed odd. Usually one will stay on the phone while the other gets vitals, etc., but he seemed determined to be the one to talk. Maybe he really enjoys talking to Morton?

~ Speaking of odd behavior while on calls, at the car accident site on the freeway ramp, since when do R and J copy down names and other info on accident victims? I guess in real life it's probably necessary for their logs and other paperwork, but we *never* see them do it. Half the time, they barely even ask the victims their names. And yet, here it was.

~ When the squad and engine turned in for the last call, at the theatre or auditorium or whatever it was, it looked more like a construction site. The squad *barely* fit through that chain-link gate. I bet it was the only entrance to the property that the LACoFD was cleared to use for filming.

I have to say, Randy is pretty good at the type of stammering and babbling that Johnny does oh-so-frequently. His phone call with Barbara was a good example. And his opening scene with Roy. (Additional drinking game: every time Johnny describes something--or some*one*--as "incredible.")

Another round of kudos always goes to Robert Fuller, who handles all that complicated medical jargon like a real medical pro. Bobby speaks more slowly than Robert, so Bobby's pronunciations are sometimes more careful, but for Robert... those drug names just roll off his tongue as if he'd been saying them all his life.

~ ~ ~

So Johnny's upset because he thinks he might have accidentally stumbled into an unwanted engagement. He doesn't understand how a girl he's dating can get the impression that a smile and nod at the mention of a wedding is tantamount to a proposal. Ah, Johnny, you have so much to learn about determined husband-seekers. Consider "Barbara" to be practice for when you meet Eager Ellen in a few years.

While Gage wrestles with his incredulity, there are two or three scenes of *only* Roy and John at the station. We see the rest of Station 51 at the first rescue and during the call to the drugged-out band rehearsal, but otherwise see them only once at the station. Too bad, and I wonder why.

Meanwhile, we have another parathion scare. Ironically, the guy flying the plane full of parathion only suffered injuries from the crash, while the unrelated random neighbor is the one who suffered from the toxic cargo. And that neighboring farmer guy... anyone notice the chest fur on him? Yikes, I've lived a handful of decades without using the word "manscaping" (shudder) but in his case I think I'd recommend it. I mean, this guy had the Amazon jungle growing on his torso. Give me Roy's more modest patch of fur any day!

Anyway, the other irony of this was that the treatment for parathion was atropine. Meanwhile, the "man down" in the park was suffering from *too much* atropine by way of daffodil bulbs. Yes, who can forget Roy's new friend Pam wandering around like the hippie that she is, quoting "a host of golden daffodils." Shouldn't the hippies and the parathion victim cancel each other out in the too much/too little atropine department?

In other news, the guys again find themselves out in the middle of nowhere when they respond to a call at a riding stable (the production company must have gotten a good rate for those remote locations for a couple days of filming). The cowboy wannabe thought he was so tough, and in fact he *was*, since he was able to expertly control and guide a horse while he was halfway passed out. I was struck again, on this 3rd or 4th viewing of this episode, that Roy gets on the biophone, and as soon as he establishes contact with Rampart, Johnny literally hops over the victim and says "I'll get it!" while taking over the transmission. Did anyone else notice that?

The off-ramp accident was a little bizarre. I found it oddly staged. The squad passes 18-20 cars stopped on the roadway, but most of them are empty, (hmmm), and there's only about 5 or 6 people standing around. We also see the engine arrive from the *opposite* direction, but other than Marco taking the reel line, we don't see or hear from any of those four guys-- not even Cap, who usually directs all the action at a vehicle accident. There was definitely a distinct lack of Cap in this episode.

And the final rescue is of the drugged-out "rock" band The Delirium Threemen. (Yeah, that's lame.) In addition to "just a few pills," the band had the full strobe lights and guitar-smashing antics, and the drummer even played a tattoo on Chet's helmet, which is funny to see. Luckily in the end our boys got their band member back to the land of the living, so that ended well enough. Even better: on their next shift Johnny tells Roy he's "off the hook" with Barbara, as she decided they should "think about the marriage thing" for a couple of months. Roy knows that's not the end of the issue, but of course, Johnny doesn't care. Far as he's concerned, as long as he's not staring down the aisle at a preacher, he's golden.

By the way, I meant to mention that in yesterday's episode, Promise, while the guys were in the hallway at Rampart, I saw a nurse with an odd hairdo walk by. Then, a minute later, the same nurse walked by again, in the same direction. The extras wrangler must have steered her and the other "hospital personnel" around the set back to where they started.

3.13 Understanding

The opening scene in the squad coming back to the station, the driveway freshly washed down and reflective for the camera. One thing we usually don't see on this show, and that's what *really* happens after a run. Like, why don't we ever (or almost never) see them hanging hose or washing down the rig? Because you know that nobody can just return from a run or a strenuous rescue and just stroll casually into the rec room like nothing happened. (Maybe the paramedics can, after a medical run.) And what about these logs we keep hearing about? Is Cap really the only one who fills out stuff like that?

Okay, tangent over. Johnny gives Chet his guitar. Why? He supposedly had a reason, a plan... which Roy doesn't want to know. Then the alarm goes off. By the way, did it seem like, as they headed out toward the apparatus room, Roy stopped right at the door? (Or maybe he pushed and the door wouldn't open? A firehouse prank, maybe??) I did think it was smart of R and J to put their bunker coats on before getting into the squad, which they don't normally do.

At the "moonshine fire," watch the guys after they get the go-ahead to try one more time to get the horse. "Right in, right out." When Cap first gives the OK, they don't have their air-masks on. A second later as they enter the barn, they do. Then they walk the horse out of the barn (masks on), but two seconds later when the girl joins them, their masks are off. E!magic!!

Johnny's hair at Rampart is an example of how it looks great from the front (bangs perfect length), but the sides (not really sideburns, just wisps hanging in front of his ears) are already getting unruly and in need of a trim. (My opinion... ymmv)

By the way, in this ep I believe Mr. Gage breaks all records in the "incredible" department. Drinking game would have to be conducted only under strict supervision, and after keys to cars and all heavy equipment have been confiscated. Because we'd all be blotto after this one.

Wonder how economical it was to have the engine idling all the while they waited for an address on the suicidal girl. Also, why do they bother bringing the O2 into the house, when all that gas had been filling the house, and they just took her outside anyway?

The bank job... that doesn't look like the main entrance to any bank I've ever been to. Or would want to go to. Looks more like a loading dock to me. Also, I didn't hear Brackett order an IV for the bank manager... they never even took his vitals, that I saw. In fact, Johnny says "hold for vitals," then Brackett said "transport immediately," and when we see the guy, he's already got an IV and is hooked up to the whatchamathingy (scope). Seems obvious that some scenes were edited out.

And what was Johnny trying to do with that bank robber? Other than keeping him calm, and maybe pointing out their lack of options. It just seems like a whacko kind of thing for him to do.   In fact, the theme of the whole episode, Understanding, seems to have been pertaining to John Gage. He surprisingly *gives* Chet the guitar, rather than sell it to him. He very uncharacteristically *isn't* bummed out or bothered by the fact that the nurse turned him down (in fact, he still wants to talk to her in spite of that).   And then he strikes up a chummy conversation with a bank-robber and hostage-taker. Yep, all in all, Johnny was being very "understanding" in this episode.   And if Roy's like me, he's a little freaked out by it.

~ ~ ~

I guess the title of this one refers mainly to the girl Ann who called in as a suicide. (Really?   Another girl named Ann? Man, these writers really do re-use the same names over and over, don't they??)   That's the only thing I can think of, anyway. In any case, I like just about everything about this episode... except for one notable thing.

First of all, there are no jackets in this one. Yay!! Second of all, Johnny wants to sell his guitar, and Chet was a likely prospect.   Is this the same guitar from season 2's Musical Mania? And what happened to the bagpipes and trombone he had in that one?   Anyway, Johnny does something quite puzzling here: after haggling with Chet and telling him he can't sell the guitar for less than XX dollars... he *gives* it to him. Free and clear.   Before he can explain his so-called "rationale" to Roy, the tones sound and off they go.

Although I'm puzzled: in the locker room, R and J are in their blue shirtsleeves. But when they get in the squad, they have their turnouts on.   They *never* put their turnouts on at the station; they always do it at the scene. Anyway, this leads us to the horse stable fire. I do like this one, and I feel bad that the horses were afraid of the fire, the hoses, the noise, etc. I do admit that I don't think that horse looked much like a "Ginger," though, you know, seeing as how it was black. But I like everything about this call. (It got me thinking though... I wonder how many roles Kevin and Randy had in which they had to ride a horse? I think that every actor in the '50s, '60s, an even '70s probably knew how to ride, since there were so many western shows on the air at that time.)

Back at Rampart, Johnny sees Dixie talking to a new nurse and immediately we see his antennae activate. Dixie gives him the full scoop on her: where she works and relationship status, and of course Johnny decides to ask her out. Talk about "incredible"... he's only seen her once, hasn't even been introduced, and already wants to ask her out. Is it just me or does that seem crazy, even for Johnny? I'm trying to think of a real-life equivalent, and I can't. I can understand being instantly *attracted* and wanting to *meet* someone right away, but to jump from "first sight" to "wanna go out?" is a bit odd, imo. Anyway even though Roy resigns himself to wait for Johnny to make his move, Johnny says he'll wait until the time is right. To me, this is the 2nd uncharacteristic John Gage action in this episode. (Stay tuned, there's more.)

Next comes the call from the attempted suicide, and it was interesting to see how Dixie and Kel handled it. Everyone pitched in, with Mike trying to get the call traced and Joe working with the *cough* "computer" guy to try to narrow down her name and address. What I wondered is, twice she mentioned her husband, Paul. Wouldn't that info be in her record as well? Maybe Rampart needs to increase the data points and search parameters of its so-called computer database. Anyway, it was interesting to see and hear the different engines and squads deployed around the likely area (Carson). It was a nice dramatic moment. But when John and Roy get to her house (did Roy kick the door in??), I wondered why Johnny carried the oxygen into the house, when they simply carried the woman outside right away. Also, I had to laugh when Early, Brackett, and Morton were calling the numbers they were given, and Morton said "I got a busy signal." What if when John and Roy arrived they found some woman yakking on the phone with her cousin?? The doctors should have been sure to rule out *all* the other numbers first.

We also find out that Johnny asked out the "incredible" nurse, and she turned him down. But, undaunted, he continued to chat with her, apparently because she *is* so "incredible." And it doesn't seem to bother Gage that she flat-out turned him down... within two minutes of meeting him. Is it just me, or does that seem awfully NOT like Johnny to take that so well??

So this leads me to what I consider to be the weak link of the episode: the bank hostage situation. First of all, there must be whole scenes we don't see, as we go from Johnny calling Rampart and saying "hold for vitals," to—literally, in the next second—the victim is on O2 and has an IV in his arm, ready for transport. It was kind of disorienting, I thought. Also, I couldn't figure out what Johnny was doing with the bank robber. Trying to distract him? Trying to help him? What? It just seemed kind of... weird. This is the same guy who practically had a panic attack about meeting with the IRS, and he's fine and cool with having a gun pointed at him? Nah, I just don't think it fits his character to behave however it was that he was behaving. So that's the fourth OOC thing that John Gage does in this episode. Starting from the first one, they grow more and more unbelievable as they go along (imho).

(By the way, Morton was wearing a pinky ring in this episode... does he always wear one? I can't recall.)

* * *

> So you think once Johnny starts talking to the guy about his "relaxation techniques" that he is doing this as a ploy to trap this guy. ... he does end up talking the guys into

giving up, but he doesn't even realize he did it. It's not like he planned it or intended to do it, it just happened

Exactly. That's what bothered me about this scene, too. Johnny doesn't seem to have an actual plan or strategy in that whole scene. During the relaxation thing, you think he's going to somehow catch the guy off-guard and get the drop on him, but no, that's not what happens. When he looks at the bag of money you think he might use it to hit the guy or throw the money as a distraction to get the gun away, but no, that's not it. Then Johnny starts talking about what the thieves should do and you think he's going to talk them into doing something that will lead the cops to catch them. But no, that doesn't happen either. Instead there's a very anticlimactic scene in which we're *told* that the robbers surrendered, but not only is it sort of a lame and unexciting conclusion, but we don't even get to *see* it. I would have believed this thing a lot more easily if Johnny was protecting the victim or some other hostage-- that, I believe he would do in a heartbeat, without question. But without him obviously having a plan, and just gushing over the bag of money and making idle conversation with a man holding a gun.... that doesn't sound like John Gage at all. This was a very different Johnny in this scene, and while he wasn't bad, he just wasn't the one I'm used to seeing.

3.14 Computer Error

Oh those pesky computers! In Understanding, we see how punch-cards revolutionized the life-saving business, narrowing down and pinpointing a former patient in only, oh, about 20 minutes. Quite the modern feat, at the time. And today we have computers malfunctioning and misplacing decimal points. So what's the general consensus on what the aggrieved Mr. Gage should do? Write a letter to Gloria Truelove. A *letter!* Even back in 1973 I'm not sure that was the most efficient option. (And didn't you love how Miss Truelove took Johnny's word for who he was? I didn't hear any account numbers being recited, did you??)

Anyhoo, back to the show. In a way I think this is where I came in to this party, because I distinctly remember a conversation here about Johnny's bill ($8.42) and how much it would be in today's money (about $45 or so). Yeah, he's not the biggest spender in the world, but a lowly county employee isn't expected to spend like a millionaire (many of whom are probably big cheapskates anyway).

In the first rescue, of Ralph Malph and Afton Cooper (haha) as Mike is using the K12 to free the boy, we clearly see his legs move, but a moment later he's all "I can't move!" Gonna hafta do better than that, Ralph, if you're gonna hang with Richie and Potsie.

When the guys are going to the rescue with the man in the safe (he sold his crappy fire-trap diner and bought a nice house instead), as the squad pulls out of the station, I'm pretty sure that's old footage of the Crown engine, rather than the new "Big Red" Ward LaFrance.

Lastly, not sure if this is a goof or maybe I missed something (or another example of creative [destructive?] editing), but at the junkyard, the victim who was pinned.... Johnny was using the PortaPower but said the ground was too soft. Roy said "I'll go get whatever" and left, and *Johnny* is with the trapped man. Next thing you know, we see an explosion and Marco gets knocked off his feet and *Johnny* helps carry him out of the way. Then we see Johnny return to the trapped man, and *Roy* is with him. This kind of stumped me. I guess Johnny could have gone for the asbestos blanket without telling Roy (and without passing him along the way), but it seems odd that they'd both leave the victim like that, especially when things are so dicey all around them. That struck me as odd. At first I thought it was a goof, but maybe there was an in-between scene filmed that didn't make the final cut so we don't see it.

~ ~ ~

I skimmed this episode today, didn't really pay a lot of attention. The big story was Johnny's credit card bill: $8.42 somehow got typo-d to become $842.00, so I can see why he's alarmed. After speaking with three different Gloria Trueloves, he finally gets it straightened out and almost got a date into the bargain... until one of the Glorias realizes that he spent $8.42 for dinner on a date. Sorry, Johnny!

Rescues:

~ Car accident in which Ralph Malph is paralyzed. He was driving "maybe pregnant" girlfriend Audrey Landers to the hospital when they get hit. Family drama ensues and true love prevails. (No, not Truelove, just true love.)

~ Woman hanging her laundry falls into a sinkhole. She gets grabby with both Johnny and Roy—and every other fireman who comes near her—in the process. (Lucky woman!)

~ Comic relief provided by Larry Storch who's locked inside a safe. Apparently he got out of the greasy diner business and took up magic. Obviously Johnny gravitates to the 'can of nuts' (heh) that has a couple of fake snakes coiled inside which explode upon opening. Roy doesn't even blink.

~ Fire in salvage yard, and it turns out the junkyard has been salvaging ammunition casings of white phosphorous or some such stuff. Drama and heroics ensue (including a bullet hole in the asbestos blanket Johnny used).

3.15 Inferno

Eggs Lupin.... with sage? Not in any rush to try that, myself. And why is Roy cooking eggs at 9:40 am? Too late for breakfast (and *nobody* should cook breakfast with their shift schedule, imho), and too early for lunch. Interesting that Roy doesn't like the dish but Johnny does.

Too funny when the tones go off and Johnny's all excited thinking it was the fire but it was "woman caught in machine, Rampart Hospital." Johnny's all disappointed and Roy says, "Let's have a look at it anyway." That's just too cute! Roy has such a dry sense of humor. Which we love!!

In the "rescue" of Dixie, or the aftermath of it, we see coffee spurt out of the machine onto Early's shoes. And not *one* of those four adults even thinks about cleaning up the mess. (Note to self: when visiting Rampart Emergency, bring my own paper towels, 'cuz ain't nobody else gonna take responsibility.) And Brackett gets called away... since when have we *ever* heard a page saying "The ambulance is here"??

In the courthouse heart patient saga, I thought that once ventricular rhythm was established, CPR would cease? The chest compressions, anyway. But they continued to do them after the heart was recharged and beating.

Funnily enough, at the station, both Johnny and Roy convince themselves (?) that they're better off not being at the big fire, and yet, when the call finally comes in, they're both as excited as little boys, getting to be a part of it. At some point during the fire sequence, I know we see the same helicopter footage we saw in Snake Bite, after the patients were loaded aboard. And after R and J rescue that guy from being pinned and they dig a hole and get the water dumped on them, the guy says "I'm not sure this is any better than being in the fire." That honestly made me LO—er, laugh out loud!

~ Cap says "go easy on the water" as they're running out, and 2 seconds later, they run out.

~ After everyone is rescued and brought topside, Chet literally just drops the hose and heads back to the engine. **What's up with that?**

~ I thought Engine 60 was supposed to approach from the opposite way, but they pull in *behind* 51.

~ When they climb the rope, I noticed that Cap was the only one wearing gloves. Really??

~ On all the calls they go to, the engine guys always wear turnout coats, even when the call doesn't involve a fire. But in THIS episode, which involved a ginormous friggin' wildfire, *nobody* is wearing turnout coats. It's blue jackets all around. **Edit:** I've learned that standard turnout gear is not generally worn for outdoor "wildland" situations such as large brushfires. Learn something new every day!

~ I love the scene at the end, with the guys sitting on the ground eating sandwiches. Yep, all dirty and sooty. And Johnny and Roy had just come from the hospital, you'd think they'd have washed their faces while they were there, no?? Not that I'm complaining about my pretty, sooty firemen.

I didn't even mention the Deke situation. Fellow paramedic Deke is severely injured and Roy talks to his wife. *ANOTHER* instance of the "Softer Side of Roy." He's as sweet to her as can possibly be... in fact, I'm not entirely certain they weren't subtly flirting with each other.

Did anyone see him wink at her? I took a screen-shot but it's hard to accurately catch someone in mid-wink, and not have it just look like an eye spasm or tic.

* * *

I hate that the writers gave her self-deprecating lines about being a hysterical woman.

Yeah, I hate that too. They gave her a good scene, with realism and truth, and then have her say, "oh, silly me, I'm just a woman!" Boo on you, writers. You *almost* had it right, and then you fall back on the lame stereotype of the accepting, long-suffering wife.

~ ~ ~

As evidenced from the title, the main topic is a large brushfire that's running amok in the county. I have no idea if such fires really were televised "live" as we saw on the show, although it did come in handy as a means of an info dump for LACoFD: explaining how they handle the fires, what types of equipment are used, etc. So it served its purpose. Station 51 gets called out while Roy was starting his Eggs Lupin, but before long Squad 51 is cancelled and returns to hold down the fort in their jurisdiction.

Johnny's all antsy to get to the fire, and as Roy prepared his eggs (secret ingredient: sage), Johnny keeps track of the blaze. He jumps excitedly out of his chair when the tones went off, but then the call comes in: "woman caught in a machine, Rampart General Hospital." Johnny's disappointed they're not being summoned to the fire and gripes, "that's not us." Ever practical (and not the senior paramedic for nothing), Roy dryly advises "Let's have a look at it anyway." We all know the "woman caught in machine" is Dixie with her hand stuck... although why the breakroom suddenly has a drink machine rather than a coffee pot, I have no idea. (The only other time we see a vending machine in there, it sells fruit.) But Roy's very sweet with Dixie and doesn't tease her, and when she's finally free, Johnny helps her to stand up, which was also sweet. Our boys are such gentlemen! (*cough*sometimes, when not calling girls dogs*cough*)

Johnny's still bummed that they haven't been called up to the fire yet, especially when they run into paramedic Deke (and his unnamed, apparently irrelevant partner) who have brought in an injured firefighter.

From there the paramedics go to court... to work on a lawyer in cardiac arrest. I always like this rescue; I like the interaction with the judge and other lawyer, and I like that they appreciate what our guys do. I think the feeling is mutual and John and Roy appreciate their assistance. (I think there was some sort of continuity goof in this scene, when it came to calling Rampart, but I can forgive that. Although I thought Johnny was kind of shouting on the biophone. Maybe he thought Brackett would hear him better if he talked loudly enough.)

But now things get hairy, as Roy notices Susan, Deke's wife, in the waiting area at Rampart. Deke's been hurt and Roy goes to check on Susan, but she's not having any of his polite small-talk or the nonsense of "he got injured doing what he loved," etc., etc. I can understand her bitterness, and at that moment she's obviously not ready to think rationally, so Roy takes her tongue-lashing in stride and stands aside as Dixie leads her away to cool off and get a grip on herself. A short while later Roy checks on her again, complete with the Rampart soapy music, and this time Susan is apologetic and ashamed of herself. They have a heart-to-heart, and Roy is as sweet and charming as any woman could wish, making it all the more curious that Johnny could possibly think Roy has no charisma. (Especially when Johnny has seen firsthand, more than once, that women respond to Roy.) Anyway, after a nice chat--and a wink on Roy's part--he leaves Susan in much better spirits, and of course we learn later on that Deke will likely be A-OK.

Back at the station, Roy finally gets to finish making his Eggs Lupin, which he and Johnny eat as they watch the fire coverage. Roy's disappointed and thinks the eggs are terrible, but Johnny "kinda likes 'em." (Shades of "Hey, Mikey!") Not surprising, considering he seems able to eat just about anything. Johnny opines that they're lucky they haven't been called to the fire--instead of being tired and hot and hungry and dirty, they're sitting in comfort at the station eating a hot meal. Yeah, he's glad now that they got sent back... who wants to be up there in that mess, anyway? And then the alarm goes off, and the grin on his face is priceless. Finally getting to the fire! And yet....

...they're on infirmary duty at the fire base camp, washing out smoky eyes and bandaging burned fingers. Necessary work, to be sure, but not exciting enough for our boys. But finally they get a call to assist Sprite 18 after an accident. When the guys get there, the fire jumps around and cuts them off, so once they free Don the guys need to hunker down until someone can come get them. Drama ensues and there are water drops, etc., but finally everyone is safely topside. My favorite line of the whole episode is after they're surrounded by fire and dig the hole and hunker in and the first water drop hits them. Don says "I'm not sure this is any better than being in the fire." Lol, I just think that's too funny!! The final scenes are really one of the best episode endings of the whole series, in my opinion. The guys are still on the job, but taking a break. They're hot and tired and dirty, but in good spirits. It's a good one, all the way around.

Bits and pieces:

~ When they took the call to help Dixie at the hospital, why did they bring their drug box in with them? Did they think they wouldn't have access to anything they might need?

~ I was curious about the Sprite. I assume it was like a bulldozer or some sort of digger or dirt-mover, but Sprite 18 seemed to have a bunch of fire-hose on it. Wonder what that was for?

~ They left not only their shovels, but also the drug box back in that canyon. And what about the squad? I guess the engine gave them a lift to retrieve it.

~ Roy had a couple of amusing quips in this one, like when Johnny was watching the TV coverage and observed "looks to me like they're sure gonna need more manpower," and Roy replied, "Well, better call the Chief Engineer and let him know." Ha-ha, too funny, Roy!

*   *   *

I agree that Deke's wife Susan was quite melodramatic. I guess the show's powers-that-be wanted to highlight what life is like for a FF's wife (or paramedic's wife)--not too different from a cop's wife. Unfortunately that helpless, sit-around-and-wait home-maker wife was the best they could do. At the **very least,** I'm glad they didn't have Susan say something like "if he doesn't make it, what's going to happen to *me?* (and the kids)" That would have been the ultimate worst, suggesting that, like the firefighter's widow in that other episode, women are incapable of coping on their own or standing on their own two feet. In any case, it gave Roy a chance to turn his sympathetic ear and sturdy shoulder to good use for Susan to cry on. I feel like this was the Roy version of Johnny's talk with Drew's wife. (Drew--Deke... if your name begins with D on this show, apparently you're toast.)

3.16 Messin' Around

Why would he call himself the Phantom when everyone knows who he is? I thought a phantom was supposed to be mysterious, not clearly seen, like an apparition. Oh well, this is Chet we're talking about, after all. And speaking of the

Phantom's pranks, this was yet another instance of "who's gonna clean that up" after the water bomb. The other day was the coffee at Rampart, and in the episode before that, Roy (accidentally) spilled some milk on the floor at the station. Get a mop, people!

Liar, liar, tree on fire... the incident is a large tree that's burning, and come to find out there's a treehouse way up in it. Funny, though, that the little girl inside didn't start screaming until *after* her mother's dramatic entrance. What, was the kid sleeping until then? Maybe she fell asleep with a cigarette in her hand? (I hate it when my kid sets fire to the tree.) And the woman was a widow. I don't think this show was ready to deal with a *gasp!* divorced woman. Didn't they have the reputation of being 'fast' and 'easy'? (I think I got that notion from an episode of Happy Days.) Anyway, if that was the case, Johnny would *really* be interested in dating her, don'tcha think? Especially since she's not really his usual type--at all. And by the way, at the fire scene she and Cap were looking awfully chummy....

Did anyone notice the dress the girl was wearing during the visit to the station? Did little girls really dress like that, in dresses that barely cover their butts? Like Cindy Brady from Brady Bunch—she was a repeat offender on this. I never dressed like that and never met a girl who did when I was that age.

So a woman feeds her husband a plant to keep him quiet. Nice. And Dieffenbachia Dude was in his "late 40s"?? Yeah, and I'm Heidi Klum.

At Rampart, we see Mike Morton in the foreground and Brackett comes out to the hallway in the background. The PA announcer says "Can I have a doctor in Treatment One." Well, guess which room Brackett *just* stepped out of??

Treatment One, you can see the room number above him as he exits and as the announcement is made.

Also, I think it stinks that Roy had to tell ant-poison-boy's mom that her son had died. That's not his job. He should have said "Uh, Dr. Brackett....!!"

Goofs: In one scene we see the squad backing into the station... right next to the old Crown engine (not the Ward LaFrance). And Stoker must have ESP because during one call, he checks the map before we even hear the address. Speaking of maps, you'd think they would show the map-book more often. Every now and then we see Johnny consult it, and in the Inferno episode the dispatcher referenced a grid location.

~ ~ ~

The Phantom is unmasked. Pranks continue, all apparently aimed at John Gage. For the most part, he takes it in good stride--even though he does vow revenge. (Note: it's not mentioned if this is the same prankster as the one in first season's Botulism episode.)

The show opens with the guys at the station, eating an actual meal, uninterrupted. Although for the life of me, I have no idea what they were eating. It was flat and circular... Biscuits? Pancakes? Whatever it was, it looked like Johnny gobbed a spoonful of melted cheese on it. And I did notice that whatever it was, Roy wasn't partaking of it. (Can't say I blame him, either, to be honest. And now that I think of it we rarely see Roy eat, at least not more than a bite or so.) Anyway, our resident playboy just broke up with another girl-- or maybe she broke up with him, I don't know for sure. In any case, it sets up the fact that John is once again single. Meantime, the Phantom, acting as Chet, drops a water bomb on him.

The first call is to a tree fire, and while it's not a huge, dangerous fire, there is surrounding grasses to worry about, so Engine 51 hustles to put it out. (The engine lurched forward as Stoker opened his door to get out; did he forget to set the brake??) Cap has the guys busy putting out the fire--and, as it happens, getting the camera wet in the process. Johnny's standing around doing nothing for some reason when a woman rushes up and says her daughter is in a treehouse at the top of the burning tree. It's worth noting that the treehouse was previously unseen (hidden by foliage) and unnoticed up to this point. Anyway, while Gage is playing hero with the daughter, mom is literally hanging all over Cap. Of course, Cap's not doing too badly himself, with his arm firmly around her as well. But when Johnny brings the girl down—and even though she wasn't apparently in any imminent danger--the mom transfers all her attention to him in a classic case of firefighter hero worship. No idea how the girl could have sustained "minor burns," but I guess it furthers the plot along, so what the heck.

At Rampart, we meet Old Bill, otherwise known as the model-rocket grandpa and Joe, the old guy who was so worried about his wife Martha. Anyway, Bill must hang out with Dr. Varner, as they both are apparently frequently at Rampart, yet we never see or hear from them except for one episode each. Funny how that happens. But Old Bill tells stories to kids in the waiting area and gets checked out by the doctors periodically when he tells them his complaints. "Just needs some attention," Dixie tells Treehouse Mom, although I'm not sure Treehouse Mom really hears her as her attention is fixated on John Gage.

Back at the station, the Phantom isn't done with Johnny, this time setting up an automatic water-bomb in the broom closet. (And since when does Chet "shush" Cap?? Talk about being assigned as Latrine Officer....) After John's soaking, all the guys are standing around in the apparatus room, but when the tones go off, we see footage of them coming out of the kitchen. (Stoker goes from wearing his blue jacket, to not wearing a jacket, to carrying his jacket.)

The alarm is for the infamous dieffenbachia plant call and its resulting speechlessness. (I gotta find a way to work that into one of my creations.) It's not a serious call, but it's amusing. Especially when Johnny identifies the victim as "in his late 40s." Whiskey tango foxtrot!!! Anyway, leaving that scene, the guys get a call to assist Engine 51 at their trash fire location. I like this call/rescue because A) they get requested to assist the engine, which doesn't happen that often, and B) it's kind of a unusual yet realistic call. The service station owner is reported to be acting hinky and not feeling up to par, but he protests the paramedics' assisting him... until Brackett lays down the truth for him over the biophone's speaker.

Back at Rampart, both Doctors Early and Brackett tell Old Bill they want to check him out, but even though that's supposedly why Bill's been hanging around to begin with, he leaves without seeing either one. And sure enough, Station 51 gets a "man down" call and it's our friend Bill. Everyone at Rampart feels badly that they didn't take his complaints seriously.

The next call is for a child swallowing ant poison. What the guys face when they get there is a CP--Clueless Parent. She's so sure that her son is misbehaving and looking for attention that she won't let Roy and Johnny inside the house. It takes Deputy Vince appearing on the scene to convince the woman to let them in. And sure enough, it's serious. Very serious. The guys do everything they can and we get some scenes of Johnny treating the boy inside the ambulance (which we don't see that often in these early seasons). Ultimately, however, things don't work out for the boy and Brackett inexplicably walks away as if he's going to wash his hands and move on, leaving Roy and Johnny there when the mother rushes up and asks "How is he?" Yeah, right, that really, really stinks.

Talking to family members at the hospital is *not* the paramedics' job.

Back at the station, there's a touching scene with the Phantom, a.k.a. Chet, not wanting Johnny to trigger his latest water bomb. He knows the guys feel bad about the boy, so it's a rare (but not totally surprising) moment of empathy among the three of them.

The final call is an accident at a dump--a bulldozer falls over a cliff and onto a dump truck. We see the dozer driver, and the dump truck driver is trapped, but when they finally free him we find out--surprise, surprise!--there's yet another victim in the dump truck, buried under the crap at the dump. So there's a search through trash until he's found. All in all, not a particularly exciting rescue, but at the very least it included all the firefighters. Only thing I found odd about this was that when Johnny called Rampart, Early answered on a regular phone, and not one of the speaker-phones they usually use.

3.17 Fools

Or, "The One With Bobby Sherman." I was never a huge Sherman fan (can you say 'helmet hair'??), so I have no idea where this episode fell in terms of the span of his teen heart-throb reign, but there it is.

This episode gives us yet another appearance of Brackett's Bookshelf. He always pauses and runs his finger along a few books until he finds that "random" book he's supposedly looking for. He makes it look good. If I were Bobby F, I'd have my page of dialogue tucked into the book so I could "read" what the book's supposed to say. (Maybe he did; maybe that's where Clooney got the idea.)

I wonder if Dr. Early felt slighted that he was asked on the boat only after Brackett declined. Nobody likes sloppy seconds, do they.

Also, this is another example (albeit not as strong as others) of a Big Issue episode. After a frustrating (and conflicting) interaction with the young and cocky junior Dr. Donaldson, Roy does what's best for the patient, deciding on the fly to ignore Rampart's instructions and go with St. Francis for a 2nd opinion. It was absolutely the right thing to do, but of course, both he and Johnny sweat it until they got their absolution from Doc Brackett.

Johnny's Coif Alert!! Gage got a trim somewhere along the way. His bangs were noticeably shorter than it was during the "pretty Johnny" phase.

At Rampart, one of the nurses in the hall was reaching up for something and her slip was visible under her sensible nurse's uniform. Anyone else remember wearing slips?? I still have one in my drawer, actually I think I have a half-slip and a full slip, kept mainly as relics of a past life, thanks to my mom.

Remember our conversation about "light water"? It was definitely mentioned in this episode, at the refinery fire. (That darn refinery... it has fires and accidents there at least three times per year, based on all the responses they have there.)

At the refinery the snorkel took our guys up to a level and they climbed the rest of the way to the victim from there. But on the way down, the snorkel picked them up at that higher level. WHY didn't they just take the snorkel all the way up?? And was it my imagination or when they were on that platform with the victim, did it sound a little like a studio echo? Not sure about that. But I *am* sure that there was the same stock crowd audio at the refinery. Lastly, I don't think the people on the ground would hear Roy yelling "heads up!" or calling for the stokes. Fires are *loud,* and with all the commotion, I doubt his voice would carry to the others below.

~ ~ ~

The one with Bobby Sherman... which prompted a significant career change for the actor/singer/heart-throb.

First off, we start with a scene in which the guys at Station 51 are being timed for donning their safety and rescue equipment. It was done for laughs, yeah, but I have to say two things: 1) I have a hard time believing that Chet could be so incompetent at getting his O2 on... he's a professional and if he couldn't do it quickly he'd never have passed the exam to begin with. And 2) I hate to say it, but I was pretty turned off by Johnny's giggling. Sorry, but I found it off-putting. Speaking of Johnny, either the filming/airing order of these episodes is off, or he got a haircut, as his hair is significantly shorter in this ep than it was in yesterday's Messin' Around. Or at least his bangs are.

Anyway, the first call is to the "exploding chimney." A bit of realism thrown in when the address given to the dispatcher turns out to be the PC's old address--an honest mistake, which is duly acknowledged. Nice realistic touch. This is also the guys' first encounter with Dr. Snob-aldson--er, I mean Donaldson. Nothing too serious this time, thank heavens, just some puzzling instructions; on the plus side, no IV meant not having to escort the victim to the hospital. Another plus: the victim and his wife are so grateful for what Roy and Johnny did, they invited them to a housewarming party.

At Rampart, we learn that Dr. Donaldson is a second-generation physician, son of another Dr. Donaldson (who apparently, after being the father of the Virus girl, entered medicine; later on he'll quit his practice and start selling cars—and advertising them with tigers). Anyway, Donaldson

Senior thinks he can order Kel and Joe to go fishing with him, not to mention sticking his nose into the work schedule in the ED. Luckily Brackett isn't having any of that, and while Joe Early might be stuck fishing with Senior, Brackett had no intention of excusing himself *or* Donaldson Junior from their shifts.

The next call is the pivot of the episode: John and Roy are dealing with a man who's in cardiac distress, although he's breathing on his own and his heart is pumping. The guys are prepared to administer the 'usual' for sinus bradycardia: atropine and MS. Based on bad information, Junior thinks they're idiots and instead prescribes lidocaine and countershock. At this point Roy doesn't even bother arguing with the doc--without hesitation he simply changes the channel on the biophone to contact St. Francis. Luckily the doctor there was prompt and agreed with the paramedics' assessment of the victim's condition.

This led to a couple of scenes of interest: Roy and Johnny in the Rampart coffee room wondering if they're in trouble for their handling of the call, and also Brackett, Early, and Dixie listening to the tape of their call. I was surprised they listened to the tape right there at the base station rather than in the privacy of Brackett's office.... anyone could hear them, and if Junior had walked up right then, it would be "not the place or time" for the ensuing conversation. Also, I would really have liked to have seen what happened when the patient was brought in and Roy had to explain their handling of the call.

In any case, all of this leads up to Brackett's decision to send Junior on a ride-along with Roy and Johnny. Although I wonder if maybe it would have been more beneficial to send him with two *other* paramedics, preferably two with whom there haven't already been any run-ins. But as luck would have it, the only 'rescue' Donaldson got to witness was getting an angsty girl's arm out of a mail box. Luckily, the alarm went off again before Donaldson could leave and Station 51 (among numerous others) responded to a refinery fire. (Was it at the place across the street from the real 127? Looked like it could have been.)

I like the rescue in this final fire. It was dramatic and dangerous but not too outrageous or reckless. No matter how often I see this one, I still wish that Donaldson would say (to Cap, the guys, or even just to himself) something along the lines of, "you guys do this on a regular basis?" Yeah, he's seen them do this daring rescue, but he needs to know that this isn't the exception, it's the rule, and paramedics perform competently (expertly) under dangerous circumstances on a regular basis. To me, that would enhance Donaldson's understanding of how paramedics operate.

Notes:

~ The ambulance attendants were wearing black jackets and pants, sort of a new uniform?

~ Johnny was duly appreciative of the couple's invitation to their eventual housewarming, but not surprisingly, Roy was a little preoccupied by the situation with Donaldson to share Johnny's feeling.

~ Did Early end up fishing with Donaldson Senior? He didn't sound enthused, and Junior suggested his father fill in at Rampart, so who knows?

~ The doctor at St. Francis must have been a former paramedic; he had the clear, monotone voice that all other paramedics seem to have on this show.

3.18 How Green Was My Thumb

[Re injuries on set] I think Randy has mentioned a couple of incidents that happened over the years (one involving some wanna-be stunt guy who tried too hard and didn't take proper precautions), but on the whole, it was a very safe set. Funny how there was always happens to be a firetruck standing by, right?

Did we all notice Randy's brother Don in this one? Hearing the voice on the biophone, you could tell it was a Mantooth!! And then we saw him as the paramedic from "95s." (Although he jumped out of the ambulance carrying an HT; shouldn't he have the biophone, and the guy driving the squad have the HT??)

Speaking of Johnny, his bangs and hair were long again, longer than it was in the last episode, Fools. Methinks there might have been a change in the airing sequence??

And just how much time did Roy spend with Mrs. Johnson, anyway? He only brought her into the hospital "last night," yet he knew the names of every one of her plants?? (Or maybe he was just pulling Johnny's leg and making up the names as he went along.)

So here was another instance of a "fake" esophageal airway... it was obvious for a second or two when we saw that Early was holding the equipment on the side of the patient's mouth. You can tell where the patient's mouth is, and the equipment thingy is on the other side of it. The camera got a little too close and hit the wrong angle.

Lastly, I thought some of the music in this one was kind of 'off.' It wasn't dramatic at moments when there was drama to be had. For example, in the beginning when they brought Denture-Man into Rampart. The man wasn't breathing, and was on the brink of death, yet the score was what you'd expect from one of those cheesy '70s-era made-for-TV movies. I noticed the same type of music another time too, equally inappropriate.

(By the way -- if there was a drinking game for leaving equipment at the scene, we'd drink a lot today because Johnny left *all* his gear in the winery: O2, helmet, and turnout coat.)

~ ~ ~

...Or, once again Johnny misses the fact that Roy does *so* have charisma.

So this episode opens with action, as Station 51 races to a fire at a snooty French restaurant. With, of course, someone left inside. (*Quelle surprise!!*) I sometimes get this rescue mixed up with the nightclub fire when Roy gets overcome with smoke, but that's in a later season, and as soon as we see the man gasping for air, I remember this is the rescue with the guy choking on his own teeth. Heck of a way to start the day, eh??

At Rampart, Roy's going to see Mrs. Johnson a woman he met "yesterday" and whose prodigious number of plants he has taken it upon himself to water. (He sure knows everything about all those plants for someone who's only been to that place once.) However, on the way to Mrs. Johnson's room, Johnny gets distracted by a pretty nurse (much like six-year-olds get distracted by butterflies when they're supposed to be playing right field). He tells the nurse he didn't catch her name... even though she was wearing a name-tag on her chest, which was probably where he was looking anyway.

Meanwhile, Brackett probably thinks he's hallucinating and dealing with dual Gages, since a paramedic on Squad 95 looks and sounds just like Johnny. The younger Mantooth (Don) still has stuff to learn, however, as he leaves both the biophone and drugbox in the ambulance when he arrives with his victim. The vic is a little girl who has a dog bite on her arm; the doctors would like to find out if they need to do a rabies series on her, although her bible-totin' parents (who are 'new' at being Christian, by the way) would prefer to trust in God to save their kid. (They obviously never heard the story of the Christian who refused assistance during a flood.) Kel's brilliant solution is to have the hospital chaplain talk to the parents, which of course solves the problem. And since the chaplain is someone we never see or hear from again, it therefore follows that his name is... wait for it!....Chuck. A variation of Charlie, a name with which we're quite familiar by this time when it comes to secondary, drive-by characters.

Next is a fire or explosion or something at a winery-- finally, my kind of disaster!! If you have DVD or Netflix or recorded the ep, watch when the squad comes to a stop at the scene and Johnny tries to get out. I have *no* idea what happened or who locked his door, but he obviously has trouble until he finally pulls the lock back up, and it's hilarious! I hope it was some sort of practical joke, but I guess we'll never know. Anyway, even though R and J are working on some guy who'd been injured, when it's discovered that (say it with me, now) "someone's still inside!," Squad 51 leaves the injured man to some late-comer paramedics and goes in search of said missing guy. Wouldn't it have made more sense for *them* to stay with the victim and have the *new* guys look for the Missing Man?? Whatevs. If they did that, Johnny wouldn't have left all his gear in the building and come out soaked in Sauvignon. Which in turn would mean he couldn't be all Disco Stu wandering around Rampart wearing no shirt and his blue jacket half unzipped. All he needed was a gold necklace.

In any case, when Tony Manero--er, I mean John Gage--is at Rampart, he finally gets to meet plant lady Mrs. Johnson. Earlier, Johnny said something snide about the "little old lady," and Roy retorts that "she's not so little." Ummm, really, Roy? I don't think "little" was the significant point that you should have corrected. So when Johnny finally does meet

Mrs. Johnson, he's astonished by the fact that she's young and blond and attractive. And young. And did I say attractive? Anyway, Johnny's caught off guard and of course does his usual babbling thing, forcing Roy to shoot him a Death Glare. Leaving Mrs. J., Johnny can't quit looking at Roy as if he turned purple and sprouted wings. "You never cease to amaze me," he says, more than once. Yeah, Johnny, you might be amazed, but take a good look at your partner because obviously that's what charisma looks like. (I'm not getting into Roy going out of his way to help Mrs. Johnson, as that is obviously beside the point and not really what the episode is about.) And of course Johnny does use the word incredible in relation to Mrs. Johnson.

The final call is the guy with the grenade in his gut. Johnny talks about all the blood the man has lost but all we see is some pseudo-red stuff on his skin, when in real life both his shirt and the carpet underneath him would be soaked in red. I find it interesting that Brackett asked Morton if he wanted to go out in the field, and not only did Mike simply jump in the ambulance without hesitation, but I think Brackett should have (and, in real life, *would* have) told him the matter involved a live grenade which could go off at any time, which might be of minor interest in deciding whether or not to take the assignment, don'tcha think?? But I thought it cute and funny when Brackett said he could use a couple of nurses who weren't scared of loud noises, and Roy says "You got 'em," and as he says it he's pointing at Johnny. I just thought that was cute.

Bits and pieces:

~ Once again we see the random stool in the elevator. In fact, Johnny sits on it while talking to the pretty nurse.

~ Brackett's tie is one that he wears again, at least two other times.

~ I didn't think the chaplain's bible passage was the best way
to convince the parents to let the doctors help their daughter. I
hardly think that refusing treatment is "tempting the Lord."

~ Anyone notice Dixie's nursing cap? It changed throughout
the episode. In some scenes it's the usual cap with two stripes
(or bands?), but in other scenes the stripes/bands are
significantly thicker, or wider.

~ Final scene at the station: As Roy unwraps the gift from
Mrs. Johnson, he hands the paper to Johnny, who in turn hands
it to Chet. Chet just glares at Johnny.

~ All the guys follow Mrs. Johnson out of the station, and
Roy's left with his gift plant; might be just me, but he didn't
look all that happy with it.

3.19 The Hard Hours

Another "big issue" episode, although this one isn't quite as
personal for Roy and Johnny as some of the others. But it
gives the Rampart characters a chance to wrestle with a Big
Issue for a change. (One that impacts them personally, I
mean.)

So, first scene we have Early fixing the squad's engine. And
that resulted in no less than three (count 'em--*three!*) instances
of "incredible." And one of them was from Roy! (Hmm, I
wonder if that was played straight or said as a joke. If so,
Johnny/Randy played it off without a twitch.)

Then we have the big strong football guy who hurt his ankle.
First he doesn't want his kid to tell anyone what happened,
then *he* told the paramedics what happened, and acted all
proud of his son, and then later, at the hospital, he again talked

proudly about his son to Brackett, but then tells his son not to get a swelled head. And this was after his son was playing wing-man and picking up a chick for dear old dad. Go figure!

In the "Brackett Does Everything" department, we have our multitalented doctor inserting the catheter in Joe Early. Dixie told Kel, "they're ready for him in the cath lab." And who's "they" if Brackett was going to be doing all the work? In his free time he probably develops x-rays and delivers preemies, too.

Love it when Roy tells Johnny to ask Rocket-Boy what kind of fuel he used, and Rocket-Boy gives a long explanation, and Johnny says in exasperation, "I don't know what kind of fuel he's using." Ha, poor Johnny.

Who knew Joe Early has such a "carpet of virility"???

Johnny's hair is short again. This episode and Fools must have been filmed *after* How Green was my Thumb, even though that's not the order they aired in.

So the "child stuck in the bathtub" is the comic relief for the day. When he's forcing the door open, Pretty Johnny quickly becomes Surprised Johnny. And then suddenly Embarrassed Johnny, so that he makes Roy take care of the situation. He also gets to do his stammering, stuttering thing again before quickly excusing himself. (And btw, did everyone notice the shape of that bath oil or shampoo bottle on the edge of the tub? It was yellow, right next to Roy.) After he frees her, the girl thanks Roy, and he says "you're welcome" without even looking at her and he hustles out without a backward glance, suds and wet arm and all. Too cute!

The squad's locked door... did anyone notice that after leaving the bathtub call, Johnny has to unlock the door of the squad? This is the first time since the series began that I've noticed this prank (if I'm wrong, let me know), but I know it won't be the last.

Last rescue, of the powerline worker who got hit with wires, once they get him down, I like how all the other guys automatically kick in to help. Someone brings the biophone and drug box, and of course Stoker's ready to help with CPR or whatever they need. A true team-- the other guys know that when they have a victim, Johnny and Roy's focus is on the victim, and anything they (Chet, Marco, Mike, Cap) do to help is appreciated, because even a few seconds can end up making all the difference. (Question: don't the wires for the EKG hookup get impacted by the defibrillation?? I'd think one might affect the other in some way. But I guess not, they obviously know what they're doing.)

Anyway, at the end of the day Early is fine and enjoying his chowder while perusing his secret stash of skin-mags.

~ ~ ~

Dr. Early (Bobby Troup) gets a chance to shine in this one. First he proves he's a Renaissance Man by expertly fixing whatever's wrong with the squad's engine (not sure when Johnny started using the word 'bloody,' btw). Anyway, a peek under the hood, a turn of the screwdriver, and bing-bang-boom, the squad is purring like a proverbial kitten. In gratitude and saving them from calling the 'repair shop,' Roy and Johnny promise to deliver to Early some of Captain Stanley's clam chowder next time he makes it. Interestingly, Roy even uses the word *incredible* in talking to Johnny, which I imagine is totally deliberate and ironic.

Early's day takes a bad turn after that. Once he's treated someone's injured hand, Kel asks to see him "for a minute." (Really, Kel? A minute??) Now comes the really crappy part of Early's day as he realizes the person with serious ticker trouble is *him*. Although I wonder if it might have occurred to him that hey, *I* had a regular physical a few days ago, and *I* have a negative heart history. I'd think the light bulb would have at least flickered in his mind at that. But in any case, that's a bunch of bad stuff to deal with. I've heard of people who go to the doctor for a routine physical and end up being admitted to the hospital, but that has got to be the most scary, jarring experience to know that you have to do this *now*, with no waiting, no delay, no chance to think about it or even prepare. It's gotta be tough, and Bobby Troup brings that fear to life.

Meanwhile, our boys get called to help a football player who got tackled and took a hard fall. It's sort of strange, one minute he's angry with the kid, then he's proud of him, then angry again. I'm not even sure why he was embarrassed to admit what happened. (Sheesh, and they call *women* vain....) I'm also not sure why Johnny rides to Rampart with him; there was no IV so it shouldn't have been necessary. And again the dad has the Jekyll-and-Hyde thing going on when he leaves Rampart, angrily telling the kid that "we'll talk about this at home." Even after the kid rounded up a nice-looking woman to fix up his dad with.

Back at the station, John and Roy are pretty bummed about Early, but don't say anything about it to the others until they know more. The fly in the ointment is the fact that Cap made lunch and it's--you guessed it--clam chowder. And he takes it a little personally when the paramedics seem to lose their appetite. Before Cap can get to the bottom of things, the whole station gets called to the scene of a kid in a rocket ship. At the sight of the smoking rocket Johnny puts on all his gear, but Roy discovers the smoke is simply from dry ice.

Best line:

Roy: Ask him what kind of fuel he's using.

Johnny (to Clyde): What kind of fuel are you using?

Clyde: Oxides of carbon and hydrogen under expansion.

Johnny (to Roy): I don't know what he's using!

Haha, too funny!

Back at Rampart, Brackett is trying to stay busy, treating Clyde's gashed arm and suggesting that his dad spend more time with him and do stuff with him. Hopefully the dad won't just take the kid to the local stock trading floor, which I'm sure is *his* idea of fun. Otherwise, Brackett and Dixie are bemoaning the fact that when they could really use distraction, the ED is quieter than usual.

Roy and Johnny finally tell Cap why they're distracted, but before they can do anything else, they get called out for a "child locked in bathroom." As they soon find out, the 'child' in question is actually a very attractive young woman, and she's stuck in a bubble bath. Yep, it's the infamous girl-stuck-in-tub scene. Johnny, suave ladies' man that he is, looks like a deer in the headlights and beats a hasty retreat as quickly as he can (with the lame excuse of getting some info from the mother), leaving Roy to deal with the "child stuck in tub." Leaving the scene, when Johnny tries to open the squad door, it's locked, which means that the on-set pranks have begun. Without missing a beat, Randy reaches in and unlocks it, which is funny, because when they arrived at the scene, the squad window had been *closed,* and now it's open. Incidentally, the girl's name was Betty... same name as the girl Johnny dated for a while.

The last call is to a "possible electrocution in a parking lot," although I didn't see a parking lot, I saw a field or vacant lot with utility poles. Anyway, it was a tricky one, and the whole station pitched in, with Marco and Stoker stationed at one pole, and Chet at the other one, and Cap coordinating the cutting of power lines while Roy and Johnny were stuffed into the cherrypicker basket trying to treat the victim. Once on the ground, everyone again pitches in--I love how they all work like a team, doing whatever needs to be done, no matter how small the task. I wonder if the paramedics ever acknowledge the other guys and the help they provide when necessary; in an urgent situation even something as simple as setting up the biophone is a help.

After dealing with Squad 51 at the base station, Kel and Dixie get the good news from Dr. Crazy-pants (that is, Nick Nolte) that Joe Early made it through surgery just fine, and of course they're very relieved. They pass the news along to the paramedics when they arrive with their electrocution victim. The next day Johnny and Roy arrive to visit Joe at the exact moment when Dixie, Brackett, and Morton all happen to be there as well--what luck! Johnny's got a thermos of Cap's clam chowder (and another shawl-collared sweater) and Roy's got his jacket over his shoulder like he's Mr. GQ. Brackett soon shoos everyone out so Early can get some rest... at which time the patient promptly opens his thermos of chowder and also pulls out the hidden skin mags. You know what they say: just because there's snow on the roof doesn't mean there's no fire inside.

Notes: one of the ambulance drivers we see here is played by Scott Gourlay, who usually plays a police officer, or sometimes an orderly. Also, the boy who played Clyde also played another smart kid on this show: the boy who self-diagnosed and borrowed Dr. Brackett's medical book. Both those episodes, the boy's 'father' despaired of what to do with him, and Brackett told both fathers the same thing.

* * *

I've had this (or a similar) conversation about this before, and I believe that adults didn't really wear t-shirts at that time (as outer wear). We kids did, but I think we're possibly the first generation to do so, and to carry the habit into adulthood. For anyone born prior to, say, the late '50s or early '60s, t-shirts were known as undershirts, for obvious reasons, as they were worn 'under' other clothing. In the episode with the parade and the old engine, when John and Roy show up at the station on their off-day to work on the engine, Johnny's wearing Jeans, a t-shirt (not white), and a button-up shirt thrown over it (but not buttoned). I think that's as close as we come to seeing anyone on this show wearing a t-shirt as an 'outer' shirt.

3.20 Floor Brigade

~ First scene-- hmmm, Roy had been trying to call Johnny since the previous afternoon. *Where* has Johnny been all that time? Why, on a date with a woman who's--say it with me, now—"*incredible.*" (what else??) Makes you wonder how late the date went, or where they went on the date, since Johnny was dressed like he'd been hiking the Rockies. (Sheepskin-lined jacket and heavy cable-knit sweater.) Roy, on the other hand, didn't even bother putting on a t-shirt underneath his uniform. Not that anyone's complaining, mind you....

~ Roy ends the telephone call with "bye-bye." My father used to do the same thing. He hated talking on the phone--thought it should be reserved only to impart or exchange vital information, and not to chat--but when he did take a call, he ended it by saying bye-bye. I never did figure out why, and now Roy does the same thing.

~ Sam the dispatcher gives the location of the cave by using map-grid coordinates. At least, I assume "grid 37A-1" refers to the map grid. Also that dirt road they turned onto is going to become stock footage, as we'll definitely see that clip again.

~ The janitor who was cleaning floors at the hospital is the same actor who was the serial patient, faking symptoms so he could stay at the hospital. He was in a couple other eps as well, along with a handful of Adam-12 appearances.

~ We get the soapy shmaltzy music again when Dr. Morton's dealing with the diabetic singer.

~ Dixie's using a green pen when taking "Mr. Smith's" information. Wonder if she stole it from Johnny's stash of green pens? .... Mr. Smith is of course Mr. Haney of Green Acres. .... After talking Roy out of calling the man about the floor cleaner, Johnny takes Roy's dime out of the coin return on the pay phone and keeps it. .... Climbing down out of the light tower, Roy sounds like "Mr. McBeevy," from an Andy Griffith episode. .... Once again, Cap and "the guys" stand on the ground and watch while Roy and Johnny do the grunt work. .... Right before the last rescue, Chet's cooking and double-dipping when he tastes: he'll take a taste from the spoon, and then use the spoon to stir whatever he's cooking. He does it not once, not twice, but *three* times.

- Final rescue is at a chemical plant.... which oddly enough is located in the heart of a commercial area. Yeah, because if I owned a florist shop or coffee house, I'd want it to be right next door to a friggin' chemical company.

And the moral of this episode is obviously, in the words of John Roderick Gage, "In business, you gotta be fast, or somebody's gonna beat you to the punch." *Riiiight.* This coming from the same guy who wouldn't let Roy call right away about the machine, but told him to wait. And we all know how *that* worked out. (Seriously, why does Roy even listen to Johnny??)

~ ~ ~

So the very first scene, we get some serious mixed messages about appropriate clothing. Roy's almost finished dressing for his shift, except once again he's forgotten his white t-shirt (yes, it's an *undershirt*, as we recently discussed)... not that anyone's complaining about the bare-chest sighting, of course. However, on the other end of the spectrum is John Gage, who comes waltzing in wearing a cable knit sweater *and* a leather-and-shearling jacket. Looks like he's ready for the slopes in Utah rather than a day in sunny SoCal.

In any case, Roy's excited because of a note he saw at the "market" (really? does anyone ever call it a market??) for a floor-cleaning machine. He thinks it's a great deal and a great idea for him and Johnny to make extra money on their off-days. Johnny's probably still 'grooving on' his date the previous day/night and not too keen on the whole cleaning thing right off the bat, but he eventually warms up to it... to the point that he's thinking of bringing in other firemen and other cleaning guys and buying more machines or even going the franchise route.

Meanwhile, duty calls and the station gets called to a man trapped in a cave-in. In general I like this rescue and following storyline at Rampart except for one thing: I can't stand the man's voice. To me he'll always be Mr. Haney from Green Acres or whatever show he was on, and the sound of his voice drives me nuts. Other than that, I do like the storyline. (By the way, once they pull him out of the cave and Roy gets authorization for an IV, he inadvertently refers to Chet as "Tim." It's sort of in an undertone but you can definitely hear him say Tim. Although the closed captioning does say Chet.) Also, the station gets called out at 8:17, but when they talk to Rampart the clock there shows 10:30. I really don't think it took them 2 hours to get the guy out.

Speaking of Rampart, Dr. Morton gets pulled into a situation of a woman who staggers into the ED requesting a doctor (she don't want no stinkin' nurse). She's a singer who hit the skids and disappeared and is now attempting a comeback. She insists she's not drunk, and she's right, but she' hasn't been managing her diabetes correctly and that's the source of her problems. Mike is polite but firm with her and things end nicely enough. Hate to say it, but I don't find this story compelling enough to pay full attention to it.

Next is the call for a "man trapped on tower" at the generic-sounding Valley College stadium. This call is notable for a number of reasons. **One,** as the squad and engine are approaching the place, we see a station wagon pull up to a stop sign. The engine and squad take the corner and come toward the camera. Meanwhile we see the station wagon is still sitting at the stop sign. We never do see it turn; it sits at that Stop sign as the squad and engine enter the college parking lot and come to a stop. The **second** notable thing is, the bolt that locks the gate to the tower is intact, so how did the kids get up there? **Thirdly,** when Johnny's foot slips and he stumbles, Randy has to give his head a little extra shake so that his helmet will fall off, because it didn't fall off on its own. And **fourthly,** when Johnny slipped, he was already 4/5 of the way to the top. Even though Roy does help him down to the next landing, it seems to take Roy an awful long time to get up to where the "man" is.

After the two culprits are taken away, Johnny gets his ribs x-rayed at Rampart; after feeling him up for a few minutes, Dr. Early confirms that Johnny's just bruised, and nothing's broken. Obviously feeling better (or maybe enjoying some potent pain-relievers), Gage starts dreaming big about the cleaning business. While Roy wants to start slow and take things a step at a time, Johnny says "in business you gotta be fast, or someone else is gonna beat you to the punch." Foreshadowing much?? Because at the station, when Roy finally calls the man, he's told that the man already sold his cleaning machine. If Roy had called when he *wanted* to call, they'd have gotten it, but Johnny told him that nobody was going to buy the machine between 12 and 1:00. Open mouth, insert foot, Mr. Gage!

Last call is the explosion and fire at a chemical company. The Universal backlot was the setting for this one, as the chemical company was inexplicably located in the middle of a commercial district. (Maybe that's why the florist next door had such beautiful flowers?? Ya never know!) And of course, there's the usual surprise of one person left inside. Johnny gears up and runs into the building, backed by Marco and Chet on the hose. Gage leads them up the stairs but an explosion causes some of the ceiling to fall and blocks the stairway, cutting off the two below. What I found odd was that Johnny not only didn't stop to help or check on them, but he just walked off without saying a word. He could at least have said "you guys OK? I'm going to find the scientist." For all Chet knew, Johnny could've been buried under some rubble. Or, for all Johnny knew, vice versa with Chet and Marco.

After finding the missing scientist, Johnny has to run inside again, to take a picture of some formula or other that's written on a blackboard. The company man says it's the "formula that triggered the explosion," which makes it sound like the Most Dangerous. Blackboard. Ever. But even if that's what caused the explosion, you'd think they'd already have the formula written down somewhere (safe), or the people in Buffalo have it, or something. In any event, the whole point of this seems to be to have Johnny go take a picture of the blackboard. Which he does. Why he later on still has a copy of the photo, though, is beyond me. Ever heard of proprietary information, John?? If he's not careful, Vince could be coming to arrest him for corporate espionage.

3.21 Propinquity

Interesting title name, not a word you hear often. But it fits.

~ While the DeSoto home is being debugged, Joanne's taking the kids to her mother's? I thought her mother lived far away and had to fly in to visit? Oh well, if TV shows can have entire characters disappear completely (*cough*Chuck Cunningham*cough*) then mothers-in-law can relocate easily enough.

~ Roy and Johnny's conversation: Roy says "I don't want to put you out." I half-expected Johnny to reply "I like to put out." LOLOL, how funny would *that* have been? And Roy with his sense of humor... he says "I don't know, me sleeping on the bed, you sleeping on the sofa...." Hahaha, good one, Roy. Oh wait, were you serious...?

~ On the way to the first rescue, the car on fire, there's a quick, blink-and-you-miss-it glimpse of the scene from The Old Engine, when the station first gets the new engine and John and Roy ride on the tailboard.

~ When the ambulance is driving along, right before it was in the accident, it looked like they were driving through a cemetery or a park, someplace with winding, curvy roads that turn at right angles for no apparent reason. Really strange. (Also, this episode had a lot of audio of tires squealing, both the ambulance and Johnny driving the squad, etc.)

~ Speaking of the ambulance and squad... I call bogus on Johnny calling in to respond to the accident just because he's "near the scene." He has no way of knowing it's Roy's ambulance that's involved, and he has no drug box or biophone with him, he'd *never* have responded--alone and unequipped--when a fully-functional squad could be called out. But, it wouldn't have been as dramatic, and we couldn't have had Johnny say "what the hell happened?" Right?

~ The call at the poker game was at a familiar house. I believe (?) that's where Johnny delivered his first baby in season 1, and I think maybe one other time we see that same house. (It's in an episode of Adam-12, too.) Speaking of the poker game, why does Johnny feel the need to tell Brackett "he'll go to the hospital if I play his hand"?? Brackett doesn't need to know that, there's nothing he can do, especially about the card game. That's a situation for Johnny and Roy to deal with.

~ At the refinery, once Roy finally gets the pinned man free and goes to help find the other missing people, he leaves the drug box where they'd been working, amid the wreckage. And it's open. Let me repeat that: he leaves the drug box behind... *open.*

~ After Johnny gets his first guy free and the guy tells him there are two more trapped somewhere, Johnny calls out to the nearest fireman, "Hey, you!" It was a guy from "12s" (and I assume a real firefighter). But I think it's funny that Johnny just commandeered him like that.

* * *

The thing that bothered me about the accident with the ambulance is wouldn't Johnny normally be following the ambulance to Rampart Hospital and also have on his lights and siren?

I think maybe that's why the writers gave us that guy, the driver of the truck who kept pestering Johnny to look at him and treat him. Once the woman, who was the priority victim, went off in the ambulance with Roy, only then did Johnny get a chance to look at the guy, thus delaying him from following the ambulance with lights and siren, i.e., it was done on purpose in the writing room.

(Now that I think about it, I kind of wonder *why* the squad follows so closely with lights and siren? It's not like they have the victim, or can help the victim in any way. The paramedic in the ambulance has the drug box, the biophone to talk to Rampart, and an attendant to assist as necessary, so I don't see that the squad following so closely is really required. Basically, it just goes to Rampart to provide a 'ride home' to the one who rode in the ambulance.)

~ ~ ~

Someone consulted his dictionary (or thesaurus) when this episode was titled, as propinquity means nearness or proximity. And that was the problem with John and Roy in this one: Roy reluctantly agreed to stay at John's place while his house is being tented. (He wanted an excuse not to stay with his family... all the "problems and little chores" have been getting him down. Well, guess what, Roy?? Real grown-ups don't run away every time things "get them down." On the other hand, I understand how he feels and can sympathize. But still, I hope that Joanne sometimes has "car trouble" when she visits friends out of town, and leaves Roy at home with the kids.)

Anyway, the first call is to a car/tanker truck accident that of course involves a fire. This whole rescue is a little schizophrenic, if you ask me. When they get there, the entire accident scene and fire is in shadow. But when Roy uses the squad to pull the crashed car away, the same scenery is all in the sun. It's a clear case of part of the rescue being filmed in the morning and the other part in the afternoon. Also, when Roy and John first run to the car (before they moved it), Roy just kind of moves one of the barrels off the hood, as if it was nothing. The barrel was marked Flammable and I assume it was supposed to be filled with gasoline, but he tossed it down as if it was nothing and as if there was no danger in doing so.

Also, when arriving at the scene, Randy has to unlock his door to get out again. Someone really is messing with him in these episodes!

Speaking of the rescue of the woman in the car, I noticed that when putting her onto the stretcher Roy says "We have to watch her back, try to keep it straight." Why didn't they just put her on a backboard to begin with??

As for the ambulance accident, I've said it before that Johnny would never have responded to the call he heard over the radio, even if he *was* right in the area. He didn't have a partner, a biophone, or a drugbox, so he would have been pretty useless all by himself. And I have a feeling that LA wouldn't have allowed him to be the sole responder; they would have kept the other squad. Anyway, I thought it was funny that the ambulance driver, played by Angelo DeMeo (Randy's stunt double), is named Hal, which is the real name of Roy's stunt double.

I thought the music during the ambulance rescue was pretty interesting. Can't remember if we've heard it before, maybe it's not new at all. Anyway, I feel bad for Johnny at Rampart when Roy leaves before Johnny could put that cream on his burned leg.

Once again, the timeline on this show confuses me. For the most part the guys work one day on, two days off, so let's say the first part of this show takes place on a Monday. Monday night they'd sleep at the station, so that means that it would be Tuesday night when Roy stayed at Johnny's house. I assume he only spent one night there, but the next day, they were both back on duty at the station. Was that Wednesday? That would only leave one day off between shifts, and I'm pretty sure there are supposed to be two. This same thing has occurred before. I know it's only a plot device, but I tend to be linear in my thinking and these gaps in logic bother me.

In any event, when Roy and Johnny are having their spirited discussion of the disastrous night, it's the start of their shift. Stoker's putting up the flags and the guys are getting dressed, and while they're still 'discussing,' the tones go off. Time out 9:17. Doesn't shift begin at 8am?? Anyway, in this episode they did get some decent continuity, as Roy's head boo-boo of the previous shift is still evident. I think the appearance of it might have changed throughout the 'day,' but I'm impressed that they actually kept it. If I didn't know better I'd think maybe it was a real injury on Kevin's forehead.

Lastly, the rescue at the ubiquitous refinery. (If it was supposed to be abandoned, why were there so many people there to get trapped??) Funny how two of the missing guys say "I'm not hurt," but then they either can't walk or say their ankle is broken, or something. Isn't that a clue that you *are* hurt?? And the guy that Cap and Johnny helped, I believe he was played by Scott Gourlay, who is a semi-familiar face on this show (deputy, ambulance attendant, etc.).

3.22 Inventions

I like this episode, it's a little more varied than some others and has a good pace to it. Plus, we get to see the guys at the station actually hanging hose!! And do other stuff around the actual station (that is, the *real* station, which was 127).

This was directed by Kevin. He seems to like unusual camera angles, such as from above (at Rampart) and from below (at the accident scene).

Speaking of the car accident, have we seen that "on-ramp" place before? I'm thinking of the accident with the young man and woman who start out angry at each other and then start to like each other (Body Language, I believe). Also similar (or same?) location for the car carrying young women that came down off the freeway and landed on the tanker carrying pesticides (Insanity Epidemic). But then, a lot of on-ramps look pretty much alike, so I could be wrong...

2nd episode in which Roy ends up with his hand on a jugular injury. (And didn't he do the same on a leg vein recently? Maybe in the car accident girl in Propinquity??) I guess you can't really just bandage the jugular injury, can you? In order to make the bandage tight enough to slow or stop the bleeding, you'd have to tie it tightly around the neck, which probably isn't optimal for breathing (duh). Anyway, we actually saw a realistic amount of blood and stuff on the trapped woman. In addition to the gory cut on her neck, she also had numerous visible lacerations on her face, not just the magic ones we hear them mention but never see.

There was Helen Crump again!! She appeared in a couple of episodes of the last season of Adam-12, and most people I know hate her character. (She's all wrong for Pete, mainly because she's not me--er, I mean, she's not the type of woman Pete usually dates. Yeah, that's what I meant.) Anyway, in this ep of E! I think she and her husband's business partner have a thing going on, so I don't feel too sorry for her.

~ John used the word "incredible," but it wasn't about a pretty girl, it was about Chet's crazy suction shoes. ... The man whose foot fell through the attic into the dining room looked like a priest with the way he was dressed. ... As they were driving to the chemical leak rescue, the engine and squad passed at least two Quonset huts on the left. I couldn't read the signs next to them, though. ... At the chemical leak, the audio people were very careful to add lots of bubbling noises. I half-expected to see a witch stirring her cauldron. ... Can't believe John and Roy were climbing those places and doing what they did-- without gloves. After they made a point of saying how toxic and strong the chemicals were, too.

At the chemical place, I love, love, *love* the scene of Johnny going hand-over-hand across the rope off the tower. That is so cool. Too bad we don't see Roy's face when he does it, but *his* mask wasn't malfunctioning so he was actually using it. Plus, it might not have even been Kevin in that scene.

Lastly, the inventions that FFs were trying to come up with were judged by the Box 15 Club. Anyone want to join??

~ ~ ~

Necessity is the mother of invention.... so when some firefighter needed a nylon spanner sleeve, he invented one. And did it before John Gage thought of it. And the theory behind Mike and Marco's machine might be sound, but it definitely needed work. And I won't even go into Chet's Spiderman shoes.... To me, the big draw of all these inventions and bull sessions was the chance to see the 'back yard' of the actual station, i.e., station 127. We even saw the guys hanging hose, and saw what it looked like as it was hanging. (It'd be interesting to see them get it back down and fold it to return it to the truck when switching out the hose.)

This one was directed by Kevin... I can't say for sure that he made any of the decisions about filming behind the real station, but I'd say it's certainly possible. I like to *think* it was his influence, at least. Also, we can say that he liked that overhead shot, as we saw it a number of times at Rampart, and even once at the station (albeit the set version). All in all, his first foray into directing was creative and well-executed.

Anyhoo.... first rescue was to a car that crashed with a tanker carrying some unknown toxic substance. Of course... do MVAs on this show ever involve anything *but* tanker trucks carrying some sort of dangerous substance? Funny thing about this one is, we see the squad zip past a bunch of cars supposedly stopped because of the accident up ahead. As soon as it's discovered that the cargo is toxic, Cap tells the cop to "get those cars out of there." Not ten minutes later, all the cars are gone. Whiskey tango foxtrot! Have you ever seen cars on a freeway or interstate able to back up and turn around so quickly? Uh-uh. Doesn't happen. Meanwhile, back at the accident, the victim of the teeny car that's wedged under the huge truck is a woman who has a nicked jugular, and Roy has to keep pressure on it. For those of you keeping score at home, this isn't the first time Roy has to do this; it happened in the Snakebite episode as well, and maybe one other time (??). By the way, I notice in both episodes, they don't bandage the wound right away... is it difficult to bandage because of the location? In order to make the bandage tight enough to stop the bleeding, you'd almost have to choke the victim, and doctors tend to frown on that.

When they get the victims to Rampart, the doctor orders x-rays of the woman's chest and abdomen. Meanwhile, she has a friggin' splint on her leg due to a broken femur... mightn't it be a good idea to get x-rays of that as well??

After this rescue we get our first view of the back of the station as Johnny checks the squad for radiation exposure. When the tones go off, they're literally able to 'drive through' the apparatus bay, slowing down to pick up the info from Cap on the way. (Cool!)

The call was for an unconscious guy on a massage table. Luckily it was a 'legitimate' massage, and like Whiny Burned Hands guy from the last episode, the masseuse wanted it made clear that this wasn't his fault, he didn't do anything wrong. This time, at least Roy answered him. "We believe you." The cause of the man's comatose state and dying organs is a mystery, and Early calls Miss Crump to town from Mayberry to talk to her (another interesting camera shot there, btw).

Personally I think Miss Crump and the other business partner had a little somethin'-somethin' going on, but that's beside the point.

After that comes the guy who was trying to help his mother by installing insulation in her attic, but he falls halfway through the ceiling. Johnny is up in the attic with Sonny while Roy directs the action in the dining room. What I thought odd here was that Roy said even if they freed the man's leg so he could get back on his feet, the attic floor wouldn't hold his weight. How did Roy know that? He wasn't up there. And if the floor held his weight before, up to this point, it should hold his weight again so he could get back downstairs. (I have an attic like that, and as long as you know where to step--and where *not* to step--there's no problem.) Also it was very convenient to have a solid beam right above the guy's head. Yeah, because life is always convenient like that.

Meanwhile, back at the ranch--er, I mean Rampart, Early and Morton solve the mystery of Organ Failure Man: he inhaled some fumes that mixed with his alcohol to a bad effect. Miss Crump is so happy to hear this that she reaches for Business Partner's hand, possibly to signal that they'll have a few weeks of bliss while hubby's laid up in the hospital.

The big call is a chemical leak at some unnamed but mysterious factory or refinery or whatever. Apparently the stuff is corrosive and dangerous and *of course* someone is stuck in the most inconvenient, inaccessible place imaginable. It's tricky trying to get to him and first Johnny stumbles and almost falls (dropping the stokes in the process), and then he negligently leans on some pipe which bursts on him and damages his air system. Meanwhile the guys are climbing all around with--get this!--*no gloves*. After all the warnings about how dangerous the place was with that terribly toxic stuff everywhere, this seems to be a serious breach of protocol, if you ask me. Anyway, the man who looked unconscious one minute is well enough a minute later to rope across to safety. The really impressive thing would have been saving the guy if he'd stayed unconscious. But what I really found funny about this whole rescue scene was the sound effect of the 'bubbling' of whatever that substance was. It was almost comical. But all's well that ends well, as usual.

Trivia:

~ I thought Roy looked particularly good in this episode for some reason. Wish the film quality was better so I could get a good look.

~ Randy obviously knows how to tie up a boat, as that was some fancy securing he was doing at the hose tower.

~ At the chemical disaster, Cap inexplicably identifies as Engine 41.

~ Kevin directed four episodes of this show. Oddly enough, three of those four are *not* available on Netflix. I wonder if that's a coincidence...?? (Note: Since writing this, Netflix has added more episodes.)

*   *   *

> So after all the "first responders" bring in these patients from the possible radioactive exposure and they need to be "decontaminated", what does that entail? Does anyone know? Do they just take off their clothes and shower? And once they find out there is no radioactive exposure they just put their clothes back on?

I'm too lazy to look it up right now, but wasn't there another contamination episode (1st season), with some scientist stuck underneath a table that they had to deal with? Seems to me it was said that Johnny got hit with more radiation than Roy did, so Johnny had to stay. Roy stopped to check on John, and he

(Roy) was wearing what looked like an orderly's uniform. I think it was mentioned that their clothes would have to be burned or something. I don't remember what they said about Johnny or how long he'd have to stay in the hospital or what treatment (if any) he'd get.

As for Johnny losing his voice, I imagine the fumes he inhaled might have irritated his throat. Even though he had a mask on, he wasn't getting air from his tank so the polluted air was probably getting through. Also, he had his mask off when he zip-lined across to safety, creating further exposure to the bad stuff. (Personally I think that scene is the whole reason for the regulator malfunction... an excuse to show Johnny without his mask on as he zips down the rope line. I admit that's a favorite scene of mine, I'd love to be able to get a pic of that with good quality.)

* * *

[Re Roy's exposure to radiation] Roy's a tough cookie. And he probably doesn't need any more kids anyway, right? (Ha ha) But if I recall correctly, wasn't he in the smushed vehicle with jugular lady? I don't think he had room in there to wear a mask (or time to put one on) while he had his hand on her wound. And by the time they got her out, there was probably no point in putting one on. He's just lucky there *wasn't* any radiation, or he could've put a star on his head and been a Christmas tree.

Author's Note

If you've made it this far and you're still reading, two things are apparent: 1) you now know that I'm a certified (or certifiable?) *E!*-geek... which is why this has been published under a pseudonym, and 2) you obviously share the geekhood. Perhaps you're even interested in reading about **Seasons 4 through 6**. If so, take heart; pour yourself a cup of coffee in the Rampart lounge and sit back to read.   Now there's even an episode guide for the Emergency! movies.

In the meantime, if you enjoyed this rambling mess of commentaries, let the world know. Reviews can be left in a variety of places: Amazon, Goodreads, B&N, etc., and you can spread the word on Facebook and Twitter. If you did *not* like this book, you're welcome to announce that as well, in which case I suggest Morse code and carrier pigeon. (Ha, just kidding!)

To contact me personally, e-mail can be sent in care of my publisher, who will weed out the death threats... I hope. That address is jyharrisbooks@gmail.com

Thank you.

May Fair
KMG-365

P.S.: Special shout-out to J.Y. Harris Books for the assist with getting these episode guides out there into the world—not as easy as some might think!   I'd like to return the favor by mentioning other books published by them. J.Y. Harris has written time-travel adventures geared toward tweens (ages 11 and up).   The first is titled *Timekeepers: A Revolutionary*

Tale. Check it out! Also under the J.Y Harris Books umbrella are a number of books by Jean Louise. _It Takes a Thief_ (three novellas) is a series about a pickpocket and a security consultant who team up to right wrongs and help people—sort of like Robin Hood, but with cellphones instead of swords. Jean Louise has also written some novelettes about two police officers. Classic TV fans might find it coincidental—or not— that the two partners in the **Boys in Blue** series are named Pete and Jim. (*wink***Adam-12***wink*) Anyway, check out these books…. (Oh, and the first book of Boys in Blue, titled _Arrest Me_, is FREE. Score! Although I personally recommend the later book, _Suspect Behavior_.)

Made in United States
Orlando, FL
11 January 2025

57170947R00167